WHAT *THE WALL STREET JOURNAL* AND *THE NEW YORK TIMES* ARE REPORTING ABOUT CALORIE RESTRICTION:

"New research shows that calorie-restriction diets, which cut calories by as much as 40 percent of your normal intake, may help you live a longer life."—*The Wall Street Journal*

"A low-calorie diet, even in people who are not obese, can lead to changes in metabolism and body chemistry that have been linked to better health and longer life, researchers are reporting. . . . There is a Calorie Restriction Society with members all over the world, and its president, Brian M. Delaney, estimates that the people experimenting on themselves number in the thousands."
—*The New York Times*

PRAISE FOR *THE LONGEVITY DIET*:

"This book is a valuable tool for those interested in living a longer, healthier life. My research with laboratory animals has shown that a nutrient-rich, calorically reduced diet slows the aging process, decreases age-associated mortality, and increases longevity. Delaney and Walford translate the results of my and others' research into practical terms that are easy to understand and easy to put into practice. This is not a rigid 'diet book.' It is a flexible program that guides the reader towards a healthier way of eating and living. Follow the advice in this book and you will very likely see many extra years of health and vigor."
—Stephen R. Spindler, PhD, Professor of Biochemistry, University of California, Riverside

"*The Longevity Diet* offers a new way of living. It helps readers mull over a commitment to themselves to live long and healthy and how to achieve it. You can take baby steps at first if you aren't ready to change every eating habit, and charts help you choose nutrient-dense foods that are still filling and satisfying. The book addresses the deleterious effects of stress that often induce humans to overeat. Forget the idea of eating to lose weight, or even to feel better. Trade calories for years of healthy living. That's the Longevity Diet."

—Bill Sardi, Knowledge of Health, Inc.,
author of *The Anti-Aging Pill* and
How to Live 100 Years without Growing Old

The Longevity Diet

THE

longevity
diet

The Only Proven Way to
Slow the Aging Process
and Maintain Peak Vitality—
Through Calorie Restriction

Brian M. Delaney
and Lisa Walford

2ND EDITION

Da Capo

LIFE
LONG

A MEMBER OF THE PERSEUS BOOKS GROUP

Many of the designations used by manufacturers and sellers to distinguish their products are claimed as trademarks. Where those designations appear in this book and Da Capo Press was aware of a trademark claim, the designations have been printed in initial capital letters.

Set in 11 point Warnock Pro by the Perseus Books Group

Cataloging-in-Publication data for this book is available from the Library of Congress.
ISBN: 978-1-60094-038-5

Published by Da Capo Press
A Member of the Perseus Books Group
www.dacapopress.com

Note: The information in this book is true and complete to the best of our knowledge. This book is intended only as an informative guide for those wishing to know more about health issues. In no way is this book intended to replace, countermand, or conflict with the advice given to you by your own physician. The ultimate decision concerning care should be made between you and your doctor. We strongly recommend you follow his or her advice. Information in this book is general and is offered with no guarantees on the part of the authors or Da Capo Press. The authors and publisher disclaim all liability in connection with the use of this book. The names and identifying details of people associated with events described in this book have been changed. Any similarity to actual persons is coincidental.

Da Capo Press books are available at special discounts for bulk purchases in the U.S. by corporations, institutions, and other organizations. For more information, please contact the Special Markets Department at the Perseus Books Group, 2300 Chestnut Street, Suite 200, Philadelphia, PA, 19103, or call (800) 810-4145, extension 5000, or e-mail special.markets@perseusbooks.com.

10 9 8 7 6 5 4 3 2 1

THIS BOOK IS DEDICATED TO THE MEMORY OF

Professor Roy L. Walford,

whose work followed the Enlightenment motto: *dare to know!*
and whose life followed his own motto: *dare to live!*

CONTENTS

FOREWORD

By Dr. Roy Walford

I have spent most of my professional life researching the relationship between level of caloric intake and longevity.

Year after year I would witness the dramatic results of calorie
restriction in my laboratory at the University of California–Los
Angeles. The animals eating a normal diet would start turning
gray, their hair would start falling out, their bones would get brit-
tle, they would start moving more and more slowly, and then they
would stop moving forever. While these changes were taking
place in the one group, there was a group of mice next to them
going through something entirely different. This other group was
on the CR (calorie restriction) diet. These animals retained an astonishing youth and vitality. At an age when most of the mice eating the normal diet were dead—a human equivalent of eighty-five
or ninety years—nearly all of the mice on the CR diet were alive
and, indeed, thriving! The females were even able to conceive!
The aging process was slowed so dramatically that many of the
mice on the CR diet lived to be a human equivalent of over 140
years, some even beyond 150 years!

I was well aware of Clive McCay's seminal research on dietary restriction, in the 1930s at Cornell University. His rodents were put on their regime early in life, one in which they were severely and abruptly restricted. Much has transpired since Dr. Richard Weindruch and I postulated and proved in my laboratory that adult-onset CR in mice, if done gradually, would trigger the health benefits described above.

At that time, I started writing books explaining the scientific principles behind CR, making the case that CR, even when started in adulthood, will almost certainly have the same effects in people as those seen in laboratory animals. We are compelled to say "almost" because the studies needed to prove this would of course take more than a century to conclude. But, as so far tested, CR works across nearly the whole animal kingdom, so it would indeed be surprising if it did not work in humans. Moreover, studies on monkeys currently underway in three laboratories in the United States very clearly show that the extensive physiological and biochemical changes seen in CR rodents are also found in CR monkeys, to whom we are extremely closely related. In addition, the human studies I personally participated in, monitored, and published results upon, while the medical officer inside the experimental habitat Biosphere 2, also show the same changes.

More studies are under way, and preliminary results all point in the same direction: the CR effect appears to be universal in the animal kingdom. Researchers at Washington University, for example, have just published a report in the journal *Nature* showing that people on CR manifest the same changes in cholesterol, fasting glucose, insulin levels, and other parameters of health as those seen in nonhuman animals on CR. The question is: How can people best put this diet into practice?

My daughter, Lisa Walford, and Brian M. Delaney have written this book with just that practical question in mind. Lisa has extensive experience with CR. She codesigned a software program that helps the user track nutrients in the diet and coauthored a book on CR with me several years ago, titled *The Anti-Aging Plan*. Brian was the founder of the first Internet-based life-extension group, Sci.life-extension, and is the president of the CR Society, a nonprofit group whose purpose is to support people practicing CR and participating in CR research.

The Longevity Diet is a multipurpose book. If you want to aim for six or seven score vital years, this book will explain how. If you have a less radical goal and simply want to reduce your chances of being felled by the heart attacks or cancer that struck many of your ancestors, this book will explain how.

And even if your principal motivation is vanity—and there's nothing wrong with that!—this book will provide what is probably the best way to look better and keep looking better. People who "go on a diet" in the normal sense, i.e., people who are simply trying to lose weight because they want to look good, have a "recidivism" rate of around 95 percent. That means that, after one year, 95 percent of the people who have gone on a weight-loss diet are back at the weight they started with. On the Longevity Diet, success rates are much, much higher. This may simply have to do with the difference in motivation. A desire to be healthy may have more staying power than a desire to be thin. But it probably has more to do with the diet itself. Instead of strange, unnatural-seeming levels of fats and proteins that we find in fad diets, the Longevity Diet, especially in its milder forms, is a diet focused simply on fruits and vegetables and other nutrient-rich foods that make sense to eat. In addition, the selection of more healthful foods leads naturally to mild to moderate weight loss, which produces health benefits that reinforce these new dietary choices.

This book presents the practical knowledge gleaned from years of collective experience with CR. It is an invaluable guide for those who want to put the principles of the Longevity Diet into practice in their own life. And giving this diet a try is something that I, as a physician and as a researcher with decades of research under my belt, would very strongly recommend. It's a shame to die so young, because it takes so long to learn how to live.

Your health is now in your hands.

Roy L. Walford, MD (1924–2004) was a gerontologist who pioneered research on the effects of a low-calorie diet on aging. He was also the author of the bestsellers *Maximum Life Span* and *The 120 Year Diet*, and *Beyond the 120-Year Diet*. He is still considered one of America's leading experts on gerontology.

PREFACE TO THE SECOND EDITION

It has been nearly five years since *The Longevity Diet* was published. In the history of science, five years is generally considered the blink of an eye. Despite the seemingly wondrous new inventions and discoveries we witness almost daily, most scientific research plods along very slowly and carefully, only occasionally offering up "Eureka!" moments. To be sure, the world's inventive minds come up with cool gadgets all the time. But important, genuinely new insights come about rarely. These new insights are often long in the making, prepared by many years of hypothesizing and testing.

The end of the first decade of the twenty-first century has seen several "Eureka!" moments in CR (calorie restriction) research. These were all very long in the making, but since they occurred after the publication of the first edition of our book, we decided a new edition was needed.

Most of the new insights into CR involve studies in humans and monkeys that confirm the hypothesis long-held by Roy Walford and a few other revolutionary researchers that at least most of the extraordinary health benefits of CR extend far up the evo-lutionary ladder, all the way to humans. Other insights involve the mechanisms by which CR is likely to exert its effects.

Although we are creating this new edition partly to share these new findings, our primary motivation is actually to provide more practical guidance to the newcomer to CR. Many of our readers suggested that we offer more concrete ideas about what to eat. The straightforward matter of what foods to choose is something we veterans often overlook when discussing CR. People new to the Longevity Diet will generally agree with the science, but are more challenged by the simple question: *What should I eat?* We who have followed the Longevity Diet for many, many years have forgotten our initial phase of careful meal planning, which after so many years becomes second nature. Partly with the help of suggestions from our readers, we have added an entirely new chapter with recipes consistent with the Longevity Diet. We have also added more guidance on meal planning and other practical matters a practitioner of CR is likely to face.

Finally, we have greatly expanded the treatment of yoga, which we believe to be an important complement to the Longevity Diet and which, in and of itself, has numerous health benefits.

May your food nourish your body, and may your body nourish your soul!

LISA WALFORD
Santa Monica

BRIAN M. DELANEY
Stockholm

PART 1

Scientific Background

1

What Is the Longevity Diet?

Introduction

The Longevity Diet is a way of eating that will radically lessen your chances of suffering from the vast majority of diseases and other ailments that may afflict us as we age. It is a highly flexible program that emphasizes healthy, nutrient-rich foods and the reduction of empty calories. It can be implemented in whatever way suits your lifestyle. In milder forms it will significantly improve your health, and more rigorous adherence to the program will literally slow the effects of aging, and, in some ways, even turn back the hands of time. If you consistently follow the principles outlined in this book, in your sixties you will feel as most people do in their forties and, when you reach your eighties, nineties, and beyond, you will still be physically vigorous and mentally agile.

The principles of the Longevity Diet are based upon an enormous body of research into the relation between diet and aging. It is now clear that a reduction in the calorie content of a diet that is otherwise healthy and nutrient rich will dramatically improve your health, and maintain youthfulness far longer than any pill or potion. This is why scientists generally refer to the diet simply as "CR," for *calorie restriction*, for it is simply the reduction in energy content of an otherwise healthy diet that produces the beneficial health effects. This diet has been the primary research tool used to study aging since the 1930s. Since then, over one thousand studies in a wide variety of laboratory animals have confirmed the dramatic results of longevity-enhancing, calorie-reduced diets. Now the results from studies on humans are pouring in, confirming that the benefits of such a diet may indeed extend up the "food chain" to humans. These results have been so impressive that even the U.S. government, which tends to be conservative when turning research results into recommendations, is changing its tune on caloric intake. For years, official government agencies emphasized that "it's okay to gain weight as you age."[1] Now, government experts have realized that it is very likely *not* okay, and may even be harmful. Indeed, the version of the government's "Dietary Guidelines for Americans" that was published in the year 2000 says precisely the opposite of the conventional wisdom: "To be at their best, adults need to avoid gaining weight, and many need to lose weight." Indeed, maintaining a healthy weight is described as "key to a long, healthy life."[2] And the next edition of "Dietary Guidelines for Americans," released in early 2005, in the words of the Executive Summary, "places stronger emphasis on reducing calorie consumption."[3] Moreover, the hundreds of dramatic CR studies in laboratory animals that researchers have amassed, as well as the growing number of studies of short-term CR in humans, have finally convinced the government to fund studies of long-term, very strict CR diets in humans. This research project, known as CALERIE (Comprehensive Assessment of Long-Term Effects of Reducing Intake of Energy), is now underway at three clinical sites: Tufts University in Boston, Washington University in St. Louis, and Pennington Biomedical Research Center in Baton Rouge. It is being coordinated by researchers at Duke University.

Long before the recent surge in media coverage of the new human CR studies, a few dedicated pioneers began following the CR-based Longevity Diet. They were inspired to do so by the research and writings of Roy L. Walford, MD, who was the world's most prominent CR and **gerontology** researcher until his death in 2004, and author of two best-selling books, *Maximum Life Span* and *Beyond the 120-Year Diet,* among other titles. Following Professor Walford's recommendations, these individuals went to their physicians, explained that they wanted to give this diet a try, had their cholesterol levels and a few other **biomarkers** measured, started the diet, came back to their physicians after a few months, got retested, and voilà! Even in that brief time, the diet had had a positive effect upon virtually every biomarker of every individual. Each shift was not only measurable, but dramatic. Their delight in the sheer look of astonishment on their physicians' faces was a major motivation to stay on the diet, as were their own observations that they were becoming trim and fit, and felt much better. But the support provided by concrete numerical measurements of their biomarkers has been, for most of these pioneers, the most important carrot keeping them moving forward on the path of health and longevity. Put yourself in their place: If after just three months on the Longevity Diet you have lost weight that will *stay* off, your total cholesterol goes from 220 to 170, your blood pressure from 140/90 to 120/70, and your doctor says, "Amazing! Keep going! I might even have to try this diet myself," it should be easy for you to maintain the desire to make the Longevity Diet a permanent part of your life. If you have become disappointed with

other health regimens that don't deliver or that have only tempo-
rary or imperceptible results—the Longevity Diet is for you!

BIOMARKERS

A biomarker is an indicator of some aspect of your state of
health. Some biomarkers are simple, like your pulse rate, or
the length of time you can stand on one foot with your eyes
closed. You can measure these biomarkers yourself, and test
your own longevity diet program! Others are measurements
of substances found in your blood, such as cholesterol and
fasting glucose. These can be ordered by your physician.
See table 1.1 for a list of biomarkers associated with health
and aging that have been used by researchers over the
years.

This regimen is not a trendy flash in the pan. We are among
those who started the Longevity Diet many years ago, nineteen
years ago in Lisa's case, eighteen in Brian's. Both of us have been
involved in the CR and longevity "movement" in various ways for
a long time—Lisa, through her writing and work with her father,
Professor Walford, and Brian, through his involvement in the creation of Internet-based health groups, and, above all, in his capacity as president of the nonprofit **CR Society International.**

We are writing this book to share what we have learned over
the years, so that others can benefit from the Longevity Diet.

The Longevity Diet in a Nutshell

The Longevity Diet is a low-calorie, generally **low-GI** (glycemic
index) diet that is rich in flavor and maximizes the natural benefits
of foods high in vitamins and minerals. It does not involve unnatural quantities of food or the elimination of fat or carbohydrates
or protein, or special potions, powders, or pills. There are no complicated, inflexible meal plans. The Longevity Diet is a prudent

---

TABLE 1.1

THREE CATEGORIES OF HUMAN BIOMARKERS
(adapted from *Beyond the 120-Year Diet*, page 32)[4]

1. "Functional" Age

Vital capacity, breath-holding time, maximal oxygen consumption (VO_2 max), kidney function (creatine clearance), diameter of pupil of eye, visual accommodation, hearing, level of DHEA hormone in blood, tests of mental function.

2. Predictive Value for Remaining Life Expectancy

Vital capacity, heart size, systolic blood pressure, hand-grip strength, presence or absence of autoantibodies in blood, immune-function tests, reaction time.

3. Segmental Aging (aging of individual parts of, or systems in, the body) and/or Disease Susceptibility

Glucose-tolerance test; levels of blood cholesterol, LDL, HDL, triglycerides, and homocysteine; systolic blood pressure; blood level of parathyroid hormone.

---

way of eating that focuses directly on what matters most for health: reducing your caloric intake while eating plentifully of foods that pack a concentrated goodness.

Since its principles are so straightforward and simple, you can implement the diet in whatever way best suits you with regard to mealtimes and food choices. You can also pursue the diet to varying degrees, much like selecting an exercise regimen: there are moderate, "relaxed" versions of the program that will still result in both immediate and long-term benefits, and more rigorous versions of the program that will provide more dramatic results. Which version of the Longevity Diet is best for you to follow is a matter that should be decided by you and your physician.

WHAT'S IN A NAME?

The diet we describe in this book has had nearly as many names as it has had practitioners. Since you will be hearing more and more about the diet from the press as research results from an increasing number of studies are released, it will be useful to know the various names the diet goes by. But don't let the plethora of names confuse you. These are all the same diet.

- **The High-Low Diet**—Named after the principle that the diet is high in essential nutrients but low in calories.
- **The Walford Diet**—Named, of course, after the researcher who first advocated the diet for human health.
- **Calorie Restriction** (or **CR**, or **The CR Diet**)— Captures the essence of the diet, but misses the *purpose* for which people would want to follow the diet. (We will nonetheless often use "CR" to describe the diet because so many practitioners use that term, as do nearly all scientists.)
- **CRON**—Calorie Restriction with Optimal Nutrition. A bit too hubristic for our taste. People following the Longevity Diet are scientifically minded, and want to stress that we actually don't know what's absolutely optimal.
- **CRAN**—Calorie Restriction with Adequate Nutrition. A bit redundant: eating a CR diet for the purposes of increasing health and longevity *is* eating with nutritional adequacy.
- **CRL**—Calorie Restriction for Longevity. Makes sense, and captures the purpose of the diet, but aren't we getting tired of these obscure initials?
- **The Longevity Diet**—Captures the purpose of the diet, which we believe is the best way to keep people motivated to stick with it.

The Range of CR Longevity Regimens

Both of us have experimented with different variations of the Longevity Diet over the years, and have learned from the experience of hundreds of other CR practitioners. Here are a few brief examples of how we and several others have put CR into practice.

LISA WALFORD, 54

Lisa's history with CR has taken many turns over the past nineteen years. She first experimented with an all-raw diet for a year, then a predominately vegetarian diet (for ethical rather than nutritional reasons).

From 1991 to 1993 her father, Professor Walford, was sealed inside the Biosphere 2 enclosure in Tucson, Arizona. Eight people lived in a virtual mini-world, growing, harvesting, and recycling all of their own food. The El Niño weather pattern robbed them of the amount of sunlight they expected, and in fact needed, to produce a normal amount of food for eight people. They all thus survived on a limited food supply; yet Roy vicariously savored oysters and champagne through Lisa's descriptions of her weekly indulgences in these delicacies. Rather than entertain living with so extreme a degree of dietary exclusions embraced by her father in the interest of science, Lisa felt it more appropriate to explore different combinations of foods that would satisfy both her senses and her body's nutritional needs, as well as her principles.

Many people are booted into considering calorie restriction when they receive a life-threatening diagnosis, or because a family member gets sick. Lisa was diagnosed HIV positive in 1985, at a time when having the disease left many people ostracized and staring at what was then considered a death sentence. Supported by her father and his research, Lisa knew that calorie restriction would help strengthen her immune system and shift the odds in her favor. Good nutrition, calorie restriction, and yoga helped her postpone going on medication until the drugs had been adequately tested. Finally, in 2000, fifteen years after being infected, she began using medication. She is currently healthy, teaches, writes, and thrives with her husband and her cat, Devi.

BODY MASS INDEX

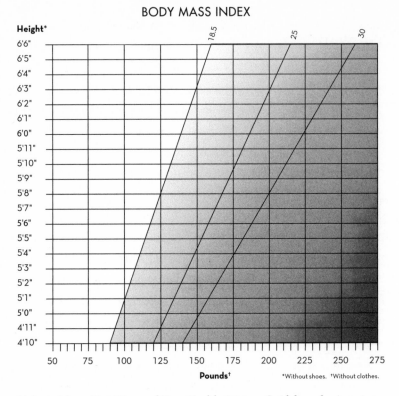

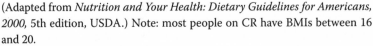

(Adapted from *Nutrition and Your Health: Dietary Guidelines for Americans, 2000,* 5th edition, USDA.) Note: most people on CR have BMIs between 16 and 20.

She was a vegan for ten years, but found that her bones needed more nourishment. She eats very little for breakfast or lunch: tea in the morning, a light soy-protein lunch, and green tea midafternoon are sufficient to keep her alert and sated. Lisa's daily indulgence is a large evening meal featuring plenty of vegetables, soy protein, and a few nuts, prepared with pesto, peanut, or pasta sauce. She fasts one day a week, and notes that those hours comprise the most restful day in her week.

Lisa's petite frame belies her strength and CR-enhanced stamina, as Washington University CR and nutrition researcher Luigi Fontana commented at the second CR Society conference in

2003, at the University of Wisconsin in Madison. As Lisa has a low **body mass index** of 17 (fashion models generally have BMIs of 17), he was surprised to see strength in a CR body. Lisa currently balances her longevity diet with an exercise regimen that includes Iyengar yoga and long walks to strengthen her heart, bones, and peace of mind, in total enabling her to live a full, multidisciplinary, and potentially long life.

BRIAN M. DELANEY, 46

Brian now follows a very simple version of the Longevity Diet: he eats whole-grain cereal with fruit, soy milk, and nonfat yogurt for breakfast; skips lunch; and, like Lisa, enjoys a substantial dinner of primarily vegetables. When eating with friends, he also enjoys a glass or two of wine. Someone commenting on his diet would probably say that he follows a standard, mostly vegetarian "health food" diet, but just doesn't eat lunch. Brian is not a strict vegetarian, however: his caloric allotment allows for a moderate portion of steak if a friend happens to serve one (he doesn't believe in troubling dinner hosts with his dietary requirements). If that "moderate portion" turned out to be immoderate, he would enjoy the steak and make up the difference in calories with a lighter breakfast the next day, so that his caloric intake would average out to the same quantity when measured across a twenty-four-hour or so period. According to research, the occasional "cheat," rebalanced as quickly as possible with a skipped or lighter meal, is fine. In the long run, what matters is the average caloric count per day (that is, as averaged across several days—a slightly heavier day followed by a slightly lighter day is fine), not the caloric content of a single meal or snack. Consuming, for example, precisely 850 calories twice a day does not yield any CR benefits beyond what a diet consisting of fewer or more meals that added up to

1,700 calories per day would produce. Likewise, you may consume around 1,900 calories one day and 1,500 or so the next, divided among two meals one day, and three or four meals the next day, to produce an average intake of 1,700, which would yield the same benefits as eating two 850-calorie meals per day.

During his first years on the Longevity Diet, Brian was very rigorous in the way he ate, the results of which were extraordinarily healthy biomarkers—his blood pressure, for example, was around 100/55. However, this version of the Longevity Diet requires a dedication to meal planning that Brian didn't have time for, and, more important, since he was already fairly trim to begin with, he felt he was becoming a bit *too* thin on so extreme a diet. Because, from the standpoint of disease prevention, he was doing even better than needed on the rigorous version, he decided it was safe to switch to the "skip lunch and eat normal-size breakfasts and dinners" version of the Longevity Diet, which continues to maintain his health. On this more moderate version of CR, Brian's blood pressure is on average 115/60. That is still, of course, excellent. Brian's physician and researcher friends all agree that he is in peak form and is probably aging a bit more slowly than he would otherwise be. Will he live to be 130 or 140 on this moderate version of the diet? Most likely not. Vanity and convenience have their price . . . but this is a plan that works for him on a day-to-day basis, and many readers would be happy to achieve his results with so easy a regimen as this moderate version of CR.

DEAN POMERLEAU, 44

In contrast to Brian, Dean is an example of an "extreme CR practitioner." Think of "extreme CR" like "extreme sports": it's a very tough challenge, but the rewards can be immense. While Dean hopes the Longevity Diet may allow him to live considerably longer than he otherwise might, he considers the other benefits of such a rigorous lifestyle to be paramount. These include physical health, emotional stability, and clarity of mind. The sheer adventure of pursuing a lifestyle different from most is also a strong motivating factor for Dean, in keeping with his visionary temperament and career.

Dean started the Longevity Diet at the turn of the millennium, at the age of thirty-five. Taking stock of his life, he didn't like the direction his health was headed in. Although still young and active, he already foresaw the writing on the wall: slightly weaker joints, a mild forgetfulness, fatigue, and a lack of energy lay in the future. Dean was not premature in his feelings of trepidation: Neural transmission time indeed starts decreasing when we are in our twenties. In our thirties, this and other health problems are of course only minor, and for many completely undetectable during everyday life, but Dean wanted to nip them in the bud.

Dean is a family man, and one of his biggest concerns when he started the diet was the impact his diet would have on his non-CR wife and kids. Dean began by trying to construct individual "optimal" CR meals for himself, while his family ate regular fare. But he soon realized that the actions required to create a single meal at a time were consuming too much of his time and energy: his family would be sitting down to a dinner of pizza while he was still chopping and washing vegetables.

Being an engineer and inventor, Dean cleverly developed a system by which he does all his food preparation in the mornings before his family wakes up. This way, he can sit down at the table alongside his family to enjoy what he considers to be an "optimal" diet.

For simplicity and ease of preparation, Dean eats two identical meals every day, in the morning and evening, like Brian, omitting lunch. Like Lisa, Dean is a vegan for ethical reasons. Obviously, his meals are not literally identical throughout the calendar year. His standard meal consists of a large salad topped with a dressing of tomato sauce, olive oil, and several sources of vegetarian protein. For "dessert," he has a large serving of mixed fruit and nuts. In the middle of the day, Dean drinks several cups of green tea. Dean subscribes to a local organic food co-op. Every week during the growing season, he receives a bounty of wonderful produce delivered right to his door.

While his friends and family are astonished that he can contentedly eat the same kind of meal every day, it works for Dean; he savors the rich variety of fruits and vegetables that his regimen makes available to him, rather than finding his reliance upon one food group boring or restrictive. His solution demonstrates yet another way that one may integrate the Longevity Diet into one's life.

ED SULLIVAN, 77

After many years of equivocation, Ed started CR in earnest just before the Thanksgiving holiday in 1996. According to Ed, he weighed in at 233 pounds, and was five foot eight inches tall ("Waist measurement confidential," he noted). His triglycerides were over 1,000; his cholesterol, over 400 with HDLs in the 20s; his blood pressure, 160–180 over approximately 110. He chose the Dean Ornish program diet, and also followed the exercise, yoga, and meditation aspects of the program, although not consistently.

Via this regimen, Ed lost fifty pounds over the next two years. He did experience some discomfort: his hands were cold, and he was hungry much of the time. However, his blood pressure went down to high normal and his blood lipids improved—but not enough. He began using fish oil, and eating some salmon as well. This subsequently lowered his triglycerides to the 50s and 60s, and they've stayed there. Still basically following this regimen, he has regained some weight, and still is about twelve pounds above his lowest weight.

Ed has varied his diet greatly over the years. However, he has consistently kept his saturated fat intake between 3 and 10 grams per day, usually about 4 grams. The program includes six to ten daily servings of low-calorie vegetables, and one to three daily servings of fruit. Sweet potatoes, brown rice, and oats are Ed's heavy carbohydrate mainstays. He uses Take Control (a soy-based margarine-like spread used in the Lyon Mediterranean Diet study), canola oil, and olive oil. He sautés foods sometimes. He rarely eats poultry and never eats beef, lamb, or pork. He tries to restrict his calories to about 1,600 a day, but the nutrition software on his computer tells him he's actually averaging a little over 1,800. He does not preplan or prepare meals in advance ("Unless that's what you call preparing leftovers," he adds).

Ed says that while he is on his version of the Longevity Diet, which he calls "CREN" (Calorie Restriction with Excellent Nutrition), he feels well, and is well. No colds, no flu, no colon polyps. No problems. With a moderate amount of aerobic exercise weekly—perhaps six to fifteen miles of running—Ed's energy is good, and his mood is good. When he does a little weightlifting a couple of times per week, he feels strong, flexible, and pain free. In contrast, while he was off the program, he was sick most of the time: He ached, he was stiff, so much so that it was actually difficult for him to get out of his chair . . . sometimes painful just to walk across the room.

He wants to stress that, much of the time during the past eight years, he did not restrict his calories with a particular goal of losing more weight than he has, yet has eaten significantly less than the average-weight person of his height would eat, (almost . . .) all of it highly nutritious. All of the day-to-day health benefits of CR continue to be realized as long as he doesn't regain any weight.

So, he's a little hungry, eats carefully, and gets a little exercise, and the result is that he's healthier than he was in his forties, and nearly as strong.

LESLIE, 65, ENGLISH TEACHER

Leslie works at home, and prefers to eat small, frequent meals. Her basic principles are to eat what is fresh and in season; and to eat small portions. She minimizes her sugar intake, does not add salt to her food, and bulks up on fiber. She loves soups, because they are filling without having a big calorie load. She never prepares entire meals herself, but does quite well between two healthy deli restaurants close by. She purchases grain and bean dishes, and stuffs the mixture into fresh peppers that she then bakes. Or she orders pita pocket meals, but she won't eat all at once everything that comes with the pita. She will save the soup and the pita top to eat later on. During the day, snacks that last include baked whole wheat pita chips, dipped in a white bean and garlic puree. She tries to eat just enough to satisfy her hunger, but not to feel full.

What cemented her relationship with calorie restriction was when she joined a yoga class. She found that the high level of body awareness and the social support reinforced her resolve. Losing weight helped her gain confidence as she molded her new lifestyle. She did not count calories, and recalled that it was a gradual process. First she cut down on portion sizes, and then she began cutting out the "bad stuff" and replacing it with "good stuff." She let go of white pasta and bread, and replaced the refined grains with whole grains. Instead of white rice, she prefers brown or wild rice. The last thing to go was potatoes—she really loved potatoes! But her sister's complications with diabetes alerted her to the glycemic spike in the spuds, and she now only occasionally bakes a russet.

JEN, 34

Jen starts the day with coffee because she loves coffee, has always drunk coffee, and always will. *Then* she thinks about food. She and her husband have eggs together, but she just has a little bit, which she puts on her thick, whole-grain toast. On another slice of toast she'll have a high-protein spread: perhaps a low-fat hummus dip. Her breakfast concludes with an orange or another piece of fruit, a small glass of nonfat milk, and then she's off for the day!

Jen eats a small salad for lunch at work. Sometimes she brings it with her, sometimes she'll manage with what she can buy at one of the small cafés in the neighborhood.

For dinner, she'll make a rice dish or stuffed vegetables, sometimes fish; and she and her husband usually each have a glass of wine with dinner.

Jen, like Brian, is at the opposite end of the spectrum from Dean: her meals appear to follow a generally healthy diet, without any obvious exclusions. Most people around her don't even know she's following a moderate CR regimen. What they will notice, however, is her long-term good health.

How to Use This Book

This book is intended to be a source of both information and inspiration. The pages that follow will enable you to tailor your CR program to your own life and needs.

Of all the diets currently being discussed and debated among experts, lay food faddists, and the media, the Longevity Diet is probably the easiest to implement in a safe way. But we suggest reading the whole book through at least once before making any changes in your diet or to your exercise program. And there is one more thing we strongly advise: **See a health-care professional before making *any* changes to your diet or exercise program.** One particular advantage to having a complete medical checkup before changing your health regimen is that the practitioner will likely order a few simple tests, such as your cholesterol and fasting glucose levels, or at the very least weigh you and take your blood pressure and pulse. These test results will provide you with a series of measurements indicating the general state of your health.

Several months after you begin the Longevity Diet, ask your practitioner to retest you. Having objective evidence of the benefits of this diet is more valuable than you might imagine. First, starting the program with baseline hard data against which to compare your improvements will help keep you motivated: you'll be working with your own personalized "before and after" statistics, not those drawn from studies of other people. In addition, these numbers will give you a sense of how well you are doing over time compared with the goals of other diet plans. But also, you will have concrete information to show your spouse or other loved ones who may be skeptical about your desire to follow the Longevity Diet. Most important, your improved health and well-being, and follow-up test results, may soon encourage your friends and family to have their biomarkers tested as well, and perhaps even to try the diet themselves. Think of all the additional years you will have together! Last, consider beginning the program with CR "buddies" with whom to share your regimen. As you keep abreast of your respective, remarkable results, it will make it all the easier for you all to stay on the diet in the long term.

Of course, even within the same family or among peers, different degrees of calorie restriction might be advisable, depending upon each person's health, lifestyle, and goals. The great panoply of humanity lives in a broad range of circumstances that are sometimes beyond individuals' control. For a multitude of reasons, people may need or desire to dine in ways that differ fundamentally from what scientific research prescribes as optimal to health; for example, in many cultures certain foods and meal plans uphold revered traditions, and it is socially or even religiously important for members of that community to perpetuate those traditions. The Longevity Diet provides you with realistic options adaptable to a large range of personal tastes and habits, and community practices. This book has been written to help you understand how the dietary choices you make may affect your body, and to guide you toward choosing an achievable health regimen that would best fit your unique body and environment.

Learning More about CR and Life Extension

Along with outlining the Longevity Diet regimen, this book will explain a few basic principles that will make it easier for you to interpret the broad deluge of information about health, diet, and medicine with which we all are constantly bombarded.

If after reading *The Longevity Diet* you have questions about CR, turn to the Resources section of this book, in which you'll find a list of additional sources of information. When exploring new paths in health or medical topics, we have found that the best source of help is other people already successfully following a health regimen. The CR Society International, for example, sponsors discussion forums at which one can pose questions about the Longevity Diet and obtain extremely useful advice. Indeed, this book occasionally quotes or reiterates material from the society's Web site. Another informational tool would be membership in a health-oriented discussion group (Internet-based or not; check local newspapers for "live" discussion/support groups and seminars in your area), since the human contact and encouragement provided by others who may be having the same experiences as you could be as useful as advice from scientific experts. Especially as you begin our program, the sheer morale-building presence of such feedback-focused sites may be as useful to you as our book's concrete tips and menu plans.

Successfully following any health regimen involves more than just choosing the recommended foods or gear. Your mind and feelings need to be engaged, too. So, what have you got to gain by extra reading and intrapersonal networking, you may wonder? Only every good reason to desire a tasty, healthy diet; an improved robustness and strength of mind, body, and spirit; and a youthful appearance that belies your long, *long* years.

How the Longevity Diet Can Change Your Life

Of Mice and Men

The results of CR research in hundreds upon hundreds of studies in a wide variety of laboratory animals up and down nearly the whole animal kingdom are truly astonishing (see table 2.1). Studies of different exercise regimens, **antioxidants,** and so on, don't even come close to producing the same improvements in longevity and health.

Over the last several years, many mainstream researchers have finally begun to realize that calorie restriction—a concept that existed for decades as merely a research tool in the laboratory—could also be applied outside the laboratory to improve the health of human beings. Even the conservative U.S. National Institutes of Health has recently recommended, in "Aim for a Healthy Weight,"[1] that people improve their health by lowering their overall caloric intake, in a diet rich in nutrients, rather than by reducing protein or fat consumption. And the National Cancer Institute, the American Diabetes Association, and the National Institute of Aging have all provided long-term funding to study CR in humans. After all, given that its effects have been observed in so many different creatures, from simple worms through fish and flies and rodents all the way to dogs, *and* there is already evidence of greater longevity in human cultures where a mild version of the Longevity Diet is followed, it would naturally follow that the Longevity Diet would be beneficial in humans.

TABLE 2.1

EXAMPLES OF CR-INDUCED LIFE-SPAN CHANGES OBSERVED IN A FEW DIFFERENT SPECIES.

	NORMALLY FED		ON CR	
	Avg. life span	Longest lived	Avg. life span	Longest lived
PROTOZOA [2]	7 days	14 days	13 days	25 days
WATER FLEA [3]	30 days	42 days	51 days	60 days
SPIDER [4]	50 days	100 days	90 days	139 days
GUPPY [5]	33 months	54 months	46 months	59 months
RATS [6]	N/A	36 months	N/A	56 months

Of the many different species for which we have experimental data on life-span change via CR, most precise data concerns mice. Mice have the distinction of being the research animal of choice for modern biological research. Thus, literally *hundreds* of CR studies have been performed on mice.

The results are simply too stunning to be left inside medical research journals. Look at the following graph:

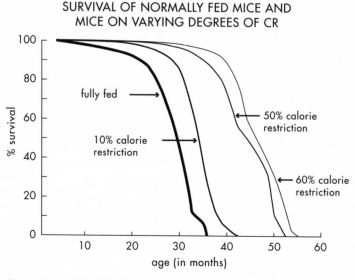

SURVIVAL OF NORMALLY FED MICE AND
MICE ON VARYING DEGREES OF CR

(From *Beyond the 120-Year Diet.*)

The above graph is typical of the results of CR studies, results that have been repeated time and time again over the course of the last two and half decades, in many different animal species. CR can increase **maximum life span** of all the creatures in which it's been tested, by anywhere from 40 to 60 percent on extreme versions of CR. Several studies in humans commenced in 2002, and even the short-term changes in the subjects' biomarkers already match those observed in other animal species that have been studied at length, which strongly suggests that the CR effect is truly universal in the animal kingdom. This would mean that we could translate the above graph into human terms, and get approximately what is shown in the graph on the following page.

We must stress that this second graph is only an extrapolation. Since CR was not being studied during the early 1900s, obviously the maximum achievable life span of humans on a CR diet has not yet been able to be determined. But based on all the evidence

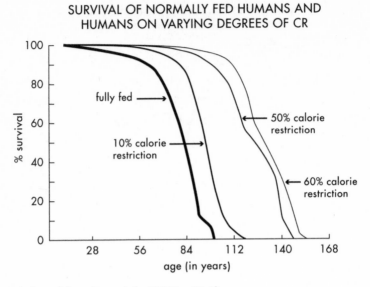

SURVIVAL OF NORMALLY FED HUMANS AND
HUMANS ON VARYING DEGREES OF CR

(Adapted from *Beyond the 120-Year Diet.*)

we currently have, the graph gives a very realistic picture of the results we might expect if we had four groups of people, one group eating normally, one on a very mild CR program, one on a stricter CR program, and one on an *extremely* severe program.

How the Longevity Diet May Extend Your Years

Let us think about what the extrapolated graph might mean in concrete terms. First, keep in mind that no health regimen is perfect. Some people have extraordinarily bad genes, or will simply have extraordinarily bad luck while crossing a street—accidents happen. But CR, started early in life, can be expected to prevent many unusually early deaths. In our extrapolated graph, we see a dip in the non-CR group very early on, when the subjects are in their teens and twenties, and the dip continues downward, though still very slowly, when they move to their next decade or so of life. If you had a group of fifty or so people, that might be just what you'd expect: you'd see maybe one or two very early deaths, as in the situation with which many of us are familiar, of a schoolmate dying of cancer or in a car crash—a rare yet nonetheless statistically expected phenomenon. As we move into the next age group, people in their thirties and early forties, another death we would still consider quite premature might be that of someone we know who has bad genes for cholesterol production and who dies of a heart attack in his late thirties, although deaths by heart attack after two score years are, unfortunately, not at all uncommon, especially among men in the United States.

TABLE 2.2

LEADING CAUSES OF DEATH IN THE UNITED STATES, BY AGE AND CAUSE, 2001.[7]

	HEART DISEASE	CANCER	CEREBRO- VASCULAR DISEASE	CHRONIC LOWER RESPIRATORY DISEASE
1–24	1,496	1,786	330	318
25–44	16,486	20,563	3,092	1,259
45–64	98,885	139,785	15,518	14,490
65 and over	582,730	390,214	144,486	106,904

Animal studies have shown that CR radically alters biomarkers associated with heart disease. Here, when it comes to humans, we have more than epidemiological data. We also have much direct evidence from human studies, such as Professor Walford's Biosphere 2 data,[8] and, more recently, the ongoing study at Washington University in St. Louis, to name just two.[9] Such studies have shown that people with the healthy cholesterol levels that result from CR have a much, much lower risk of cardiovascular disease. Thus, the person in the non-CR group who dies of a heart attack at age forty or so would very likely live much longer—perhaps an additional two or three or even more decades—on even a relatively mild CR program.

We know also that CR dramatically reduces the incidence of cancer in laboratory animals,[10] and evidence has been mounting that CR, not surprisingly, reduces cancer risk in humans as well.[11] Thus, it's not at all unrealistic to suppose that CR, whether mild or severe, may prevent early deaths from cancer, or may at least radically push it back, as suggested by the extrapolated graph for human life expectancy.

As we follow our extrapolated graph over to the right, we see many more people in the non-CR group dying in their fifties and early sixties—and even a few in the mild CR group, as well, bearing out animal-study results that CR in its milder forms is not nearly as beneficial as a more stringent program. Once we get to the age of sixty-five or seventy, people in the non-CR group begin to dwindle dramatically, as disease strikes or organs fail. If human life expectancy indeed follows that of animals placed on a CR diet, we would expect the threshold of what we now consider elderly to be pushed back nearly fifteen years for the group of people on the mild CR regimen, and that it would be pushed back even more for the subjects on rigorous CR.

And, as we move even further to the right on the timeline, we see that very few of the non-CR group are likely to be alive in their nineties. However, most of the mild-CR group will still be around then, as will the vast majority of the rigorous CR groups.

So what, then, is the ultimate effect of CR? Calorie restriction shifts the survival curve to the right, and it does so in such a way that *everything* is pushed to the right. People on CR will not become senile and crippled at the same age as others, and then be forced to live an extra few decades in this state of decrepitude. Quite the contrary; CR promises that *youthfulness itself* will be preserved. Thus, for the group on more rigorous CR programs, the cycle of life and death would look very different indeed from what we picture as the normal life cycle. If you go on even a moderate CR program, you can expect to live, on average, at least a decade longer than you otherwise would—and perhaps several decades longer, if cancer or a stroke is averted. And it's not just that your life span is extended, your **youth span** will also be extended. Aged laboratory rats[12] and mice[13] on CR run mazes just as quickly and intelligently as they did when they were in the equivalent of their "teens." They also have sex at an age when the animals in their studies' **control group**—those creatures that, given the mortality of non-CR rodents, are lucky enough still to be alive—don't even remember what sex is.

From the Lab to Your Life: CR Research Through the Ages

Prehistory

The notion that restricting one's diet could be salubrious in various ways is actually an ancient one. In the Middle Ages, for example, it was thought that tumors could be eliminated via restricted eating: Both the tumor and the body need food to thrive, but the body, being more virtuous, would survive a reduction in food longer than a malignant—and therefore evil—tumor, and thus the tumor would die before the body would. (Do not try this at home!)

So went the reasoning. At the beginning of the last century, a slightly more biologically enlightened version of this line of thought led to some scientific studies revealing a correlation between food consumption and tumor growth. As early as 1909, for example, it was shown by Carlo Moreschi, an Italian immunology researcher, that tumors transplanted into underfed mice did not grow as quickly as tumors transplanted into normally fed mice.[14] Over the next ten or so years, the development of tumors itself was shown to be to suppressed in underfed lab rodents.

Although it is true that most types of cancer become more prevalent with age, establishing a relation between cancer growth and food intake is not the same as establishing a relation between rate of aging and food intake. That latter relationship only began to be explored two decades later, and even then partly as an unintended consequence of a Cornell University cancer researcher's experiment.

The Modern Period of CR Research

Clive McCay, a researcher at Cornell University, was interested in the long-term effects of stunted growth upon mice, which in a study in the mid-1930s he induced via a drastic reduction in the lab animals' food intake.[15] A completely unexpected finding was that the rodents lived around a third longer than rodents on a normal lab diet! No one knew what to make of this finding, though some researchers tried to figure out what the crucial factor was—a particular component of the diet, or the mere quantity of food, or the total energy content of the laboratory meals. It was shown in the 1940s that it was indeed the energy content—which is to say, the caloric content—alone that made the difference. Indeed, by reducing the energy content only, and not any other components of the diet (such as critical vitamins and minerals), the benefits were even greater.

Despite that important breakthrough, little CR research was done until the 1970s, when the modern period of research into this regimen began. Knowledge of molecular biology had developed to the point where it was possible to investigate how CR exerted its effect. Over the next decades, CR research evolved into the standard, primary tool for investigating the fundamental mechanisms of aging, because it quickly emerged that calorie restriction is the only intervention that retards the rate at which organisms age. Understanding how and under what conditions CR works in laboratory animals has thus been viewed as tantamount to understanding the aging process itself. And because no other reproducible and verified means of appreciably slowing the aging process has yet been discovered, CR has, since the 1970s, remained the primary laboratory model for understanding the mechanism, or more likely mechanisms, of aging in laboratory animals.

The general research strategy is not complicated or overly technical. One approach is the following: A researcher first selects one of the myriad differences between CR animals and normally fed animals. He or she then tries to elicit the one change, be it a hormone that is expressed at a higher or lower level in CR animals, or even a particular gene whose function is not yet known, which is expressed at a different level in animals on CR. Then, the researcher tries to see whether the alteration of this one factor in normally fed animals can elicit the CR effect, or, conversely, whether an attempt to suppress this change in animals on CR might abolish the CR effect. For example, animals on CR typically have lower body temperatures than do their non-CR control group. Professor Roy Walford, along with some Japanese colleagues, showed that artificially raising the body temperature of animals on CR abolished at least certain aspects of the CR effect.[16] This suggested that this one change, a lowered body temperature, might be fundamental to the beneficial effects of the diet. The next step would be to see what happens when we lower body temperature in animals not on CR. Interestingly, tentative research results show that lowering body temperature can indeed increase longevity somewhat, though not as much as strict CR.[17]

The most recent CR studies follow this same pattern, and scientists appear to be getting very close to understanding how CR works. Research at Brown University, Harvard University, and MIT has shown that forced expression of a particular gene can actually elicit the CR effect, or at least aspects of the CR effect, in yeast and fruit flies. This change in gene expression, more than hormones or body temperature, appears to be an essential factor, if not *the* essential factor, in the host of changes that lead to the greatly improved health seen in laboratory animals on CR. For more about this exciting new research, see chapter 4.

For now, let us summarize what we know about the consequences of CR in laboratory animals:

How CR Affects Your Health

CR produces a wide variety of positive effects upon laboratory animals. Many of these benefits have actually been confirmed, in short-term studies, in humans as well.

Improved Insulin Sensitivity

Insulin is a hormone secreted by the pancreas that enables your cells to use their most important fuel, glucose. As we age, cells tend to become less responsive to insulin. This leads to unnecessarily high levels of glucose, which can lead to type 2 diabetes, and maybe even accelerated aging.

The effect of CR in lab animals on insulin sensitivity is one of the most well-documented CR research findings. One of Professor Walford's contemporaries, Edward J. Masoro, of the University of Texas Health Science Center in San Antonio, was one of the first to investigate the mechanism of the dramatic effect of CR on the age-associated decrease in insulin sensitivity.[18] Many others have expanded on this work.[19]

The data from the long-term studies of CR in nonhuman primates have been consistent with the findings in rodents. In the NIA (National Institute on Aging) Primate Study, the monkeys on CR have dramatically lower circulating insulin levels, which we know is an excellent measure of insulin sensitivity. (The more sensitive your cells are to insulin, the less your body needs to secrete insulin into the blood.)[20]

And countless studies of short-term CR in overweight humans have shown conclusively that insulin sensitivity increases on CR.[21] Although we don't yet have long-term data on CR in people who are thin to begin with, those who already have type 2 diabetes can probably even improve their glucose metabolism with CR. The American Diabetes Association has begun stressing that reducing energy intake, as part of a comprehensive program of diabetes management, can improve insulin resistance in diabetics.[22]

Even a conservative physician with no awareness of CR would agree that CR will most likely reduce your chances of developing type 2 diabetes, and, if you already are "prediabetic," CR will probably halt the march toward full-blown diabetes.[23]

Lower Average Circulating Levels of Glucose

This change is, of course, directly connected to insulin sensitivity. The rodent studies show lowered levels of circulating glucose, just as they show lowered levels of circulating insulin, since the two go hand in hand. But in addition to being correlated with lowered insulin, a lowered glucose level is a good thing in and of itself.

Glucose is your body's primary liquid fuel. Like your car's gasoline, it is an "energetic" chemical that can damage what it comes into contact with (see chapter 4 for more about this effect of glucose). In brief, superfluous glucose will needlessly harm the molecules, cells, and tissues of your body. According to many theories of aging, this damage may well be a significant cause of aging. Thus, all your tissues, from brain tissue to skin tissue, will benefit from lower levels of circulating glucose in your blood: just enough to keep your body running smoothly, without "spills."

Increased Maintenance of DNA

DNA (deoxyribonucleic acid) is the extremely long, intricate, fragile molecule that constitutes your body's blueprint. The design specs encoded in your DNA determine most of your biological characteristics as you grow into an adult, but they also guide ongoing repair and maintenance during your many (we hope!) decades of adult life. As we age our DNA becomes damaged, and not all of that damage can be repaired. This deterioration of your DNA slowly results in progressively worse functionality at all levels: your cells, organs, and your whole body.

The earliest studies of CR in laboratory animals could not measure the ability of CR to protect DNA against age-associated damage, since DNA hadn't even been discovered yet! But starting in the mid-1980s and early 1990s, new techniques made it possible to show that DNA damage is reduced in laboratory animals on CR,[24] although, not surprisingly, the effect is greater on DNA involved in the use of energy.[25] Interestingly, it isn't simply that DNA damage is reduced. There is an actual increase in DNA *repair*.[26]

Studies of the effect of CR on DNA damage in humans are ongoing, though even now, in 2010, we have substantial evidence that CR in humans reduces DNA damage.[27] In addition, although studies on the reduction of obesity are not the same as CR studies in the non-obese, it is worth noting that several weight-loss studies have shown that telomere length of at least some cells increases when the obese go on a calorically restricted diet.[28] Telomeres are the "caps" on the ends of DNA strands. When these caps get too short, the DNA strands become unstable.

Whether or not damage to DNA has anything to do with aging per se, keeping your DNA stable and intact is a good survival strategy! Changes in cellular DNA are implicated in many diseases, above all cancer.

Reduction in Expression of Oncogenes

On a CR regimen, you can expect that *oncogenes*—genes that lead to abnormal, unnecessary cell proliferation (which is all cancer really is)—will be less likely to be "switched on." This effect is very well established in laboratory mice.[29]

There is considerable epidemiological evidence that CR in humans reduces cancer risk, and, amazingly enough, there is even evidence that mere "FR"—indiscriminate restriction of food, not a targeted restriction of calories in an otherwise healthy diet—reduces cancer risk.[30] Thus, when a proper CR program is instituted, we might expect an even greater reduction in risk of cancer.

Reduced Decline in Sexual Activity with Age

The sexual activity of laboratory animals on an extreme CR regimen actually decreases a bit in their younger years. This is consistent with theories of why CR would have evolved in the first place: Resources get shifted away from reproduction and growth, and moved toward repair and maintenance. But in animals on CR, sexuality does not decrease with age at the same rate as it does in their control group.[31] In fact, this was first noted over fifty years ago in studies by Maurice B. Visscher at the University of Minnesota.[32]

As Professor Walford noted in *Maximum Life Span,* there are astonishing studies showing that laboratory animals on CR not only still have sex and otherwise display sexual interest at an age beyond that of animals in the non-CR group that have died, but they can actually become pregnant and give birth to healthy babies when *all* of the control animals are dead![33]

Moreover, CR actually increases follicular reserves—meaning, in human terms, that menopause could be postponed by many years.[34]

Lowered Blood Pressure

This is of course good news for those of you who are worried about stroke or embolisms. This is also, by the way, something you can easily measure yourself at one of those blood pressure machines that many pharmacies and health-fair clinics provide for public use. Take advantage of these services. Again, hard evidence of your progress will increase your motivation.

Reduced Risk of Arthritis

Arthritis may not be life threatening—at least not while you're still in midlife—but it is extremely painful and restrictive. We know several artists and musicians who, only in their forties and fifties, will soon have to stop practicing their art because of this condition. In the lab, CR has been demonstrated to greatly delay the onset of arthritis.[35]

Improved Mental Functioning

This is a lab finding that is perhaps most important to keep in mind if you're worried about CR simply prolonging the decrepit phase of old age. It most certainly does not—it prolongs and even restores youth, in many ways. That a mouse which in human years would be over one hundred years old can zip through a maze with the problem-solving skills of a young adult rodent may seem incredible, but this phenomenon has been documented repeatedly in research studies. The ability of calorie restriction to maintain youthful mental functioning is believed to be the beneficial result of a very straightforward effect already discussed: because it strengthens and repairs the body's cells in general, CR prevents the brain cell death that normally occurs with age.[36]

The 2004 Washington University CR Study

Calorie restriction has moved far beyond the laboratory, and into layman practice. This process accelerated in 2004 because of the dramatic study published by a group at the Washington University in St. Louis (WUSTL). The 2004 WUSTL study presented powerful evidence of the dramatic results of long-term CR in humans. Again, we lack mortality data because, for these subjects, that material will not be assessed conclusively for many decades to come. But the study clearly indicated positive shifts in those biomarkers that are associated with disease risk and that are thought to be associated with rate of aging. Human CR studies published since then, by the group at WUSTL and others, have all confirmed what Roy Walford and a few pioneers have suspected for several decades: CR in humans dramatically improves markers of health. We will discuss the most recent findings in chapter 4.

The following table appeared in the very first research paper published by the WUSTL group concerning this groundbreaking discovery:

TABLE 2.3

Parameter	VALUE		P value
	CR (n = 18)	Controls (n = 18)	
Tchol, mg/dl	158 ± 39	205 ± 40	0.001
LDL-C, mg/dl	86 ± 28	127 ± 35	0.0001
HDL-C, mg/dl	63 ± 19	48 ± 11	0.006
Tchol/HDL-C ratio	2.6 ± 0.5	4.5 ± 1.3	0.0001
TG, mg/dl	48 ± 15	147 ± 89	0.0001
TG/HDL-C ratio	0.8 ± 0.3	3.5 ± 2.8	0.0001
Systolic BP, mmHg	99 ± 10	129 ± 13	0.0001
Diastolic BP, mmHg	61 ± 6	79 ± 7	0.0001
Fasting glucose, mg/dl	81 ± 7	95 ± 8	0.0001
Fasting insulin, mIU/ml	1.4 ± 0.8	5.1 ± 2	0.0001
Hs-CRP, µg/ml	0.3 ± 0.2	1.6 ± 2.2	0.001

Values are means ± SD. IU, international unit; Hs-CRP, high-sensitivity CRP; 1 mmHg = 133 Pa.
(From *Proceedings of the National Academy of Sciences of the United States of America*.[37])
Key to some of the abbreviations in the table:
Tchol = total cholesterol
TG = triglycerides
Systolic BP = blood pressure when the heart pumps, e.g., the 120 in 120/80
Diastolic BP = blood pressure between heart beats, e.g., the 80 in 120/80
Hs-CRP = high-sensitivity C-reactive protein, a protein that is a marker of inflammation
P value = a measure of the probability that the differences observed between the group on CR and the non-CR group occurred by chance
These are extremely low *P* values for a medical study.

The next time you go for a medical exam, bring this book with you and show your health practitioner that table. Tell her (or him) to go to a medical library and look at the actual research paper in which the table appears. Encourage her, while she is at the medical library, to look at all the other CR research that's been done. Once she will have finished reading, she will understand why there's nothing surprising, wrong, or faked about the numbers in the WUSTL paper. These kinds of impressive results are supported by all CR studies in lab animals, all shorter-term CR studies in humans, and indeed all theories of aging.

Based upon the numbers in the WUSTL report, your health practitioner would surely agree that the people on CR have, on average, a much lower risk of getting cardiovascular disease, a much lower risk of stroke, and a lower risk of arthritis, and that their risk of type 2 diabetes couldn't possibly be much lower.

So, What's the Catch?

Q: Wait a minute, this sounds too good to be true. By simply reducing my calories, I can radically reduce my chances of getting cancer, heart disease, stroke, type 2 diabetes, and more, even slow my aging process—and live decades longer than my parents and grandparents? There's got to be a catch, right?

Well, that depends on you.

No serious scientist or physician who has taken the time to review the scientific basis for the Longevity Diet can deny its benefits. The documented results of CR research are more solid than many quasi-scientific claims about the relationship of diet, health, and longevity. But many health professionals do tell us this: "It's too hard for most people, because they'll be too hungry."

Here, it is vital to distinguish between a need for missing essential nutrients, and what most people generally *perceive* as a need to eat: a desire for food, regardless of whether the body has in fact been adequately fed. Indeed, all too often what is interpreted as hunger is merely the habit of eating automatically based upon external factors such as the setting sun or hour, as in, "It's noon, therefore I must eat lunch" or "I'm about to seat myself in a movie theater, therefore I need to buy popcorn."

The sudden adoption of an extreme version of the diet (or any diet in which particular foods are eliminated) may well produce, as a side effect, the *perception* that one "must" eat more. This is not at all surprising: at the beginning of the regimen, of course you'll be very aware that you are eating less than what you have grown accustomed to; furthermore, it takes time for a body that is used to processing high levels of sugar, animal proteins, or fat to adjust itself to receiving less. This is not what many would call "true hunger"; rather, it is your body's confused way of signaling that its internal chemistry has been changed. Hang in there! Eventually, you will forget your old eating habits and, if you're like most CR followers, you will soon no longer feel that you are "missing" something on the Longevity Diet; meanwhile, trust that your metabolism will learn to feel sated by the correct amounts of the nutrients it needs to run, and will stop signaling you so urgently for more.

If you experience hunger, try drinking a non- or low-calorie beverage, such as sugarless tea or even just water. Diverting yourself with activities that hold your attention or busy your hands is another way to keep control. Do whatever you can to ignore those external markers that tell you it's time for a meal or snack. Instead, listen to your body, and that includes listening to its silence—if you *don't feel hungry,* you don't need to eat! Although you may find this hard to believe, some people who are not even trying to diet can become so wrapped up in work or other activities that they entirely forget to stop for lunch or dinner . . . they've technically missed a meal, yet don't "miss" it at all. Even a deliberate all-day fast becomes easier if you plan other activities for the day than watching the clock.

Here's what a few people who have been on CR say about hunger:

BRIAN M. DELANEY

When I was on a more extreme version of the Longevity Diet than I'm on now, I was certainly hungry. I am one of those unlucky people who suffers from extreme hunger when I haven't eaten for a few hours. My body tells me to stuff my face. A lot.

Still, after a while, the hunger lessened significantly. Partly this is because I knew CR was changing my life dramatically for the good. This made me feel better, and I was more productive, more excited about what I was doing, and thus, after a few months, I didn't even think about the hunger very often. Mind you, I was on very severe CR. I'm around five foot eleven, and by that point I weighed only 129 pounds. This was, for someone who ate constantly while growing up, an amazing achievement. And, of course, that is a case of the sort of extreme results that many people may not even be interested in achieving. The knowledge that I was eating astonishingly well made the hunger I did experience somehow "part of the whole package" of eating for excellent health in a culture that tells us to do just the opposite.

Now, on my somewhat milder, "skip lunch" version of the Longevity Diet, I may sometimes feel hungry during the mid to late afternoon, once my breakfast calories have been digested. However, as had occurred before once my body had adjusted to a much lower caloric intake, I generally don't even think about it. If I happen to be in a boring phase of a work project, though, I certainly will notice the body chemical kick-in of hunger in midafternoon. But then I just think: this means my stomach is empty, my glucose levels are low, my body has learned how to use glucose very efficiently (which is probably why I feel energetic, despite the low glucose levels), and my body is aging more slowly.

LISA WALFORD

I have always been a very slow eater. I savor every bite, but this does not mean that I take long lunch breaks or that I eat less food! As a consequence, my meals feel filling. I drink lime-flavored mineral water and green tea throughout the day, which takes care of any oral urges. I am also a grazer, so I nibble on a small amount of nuts or fruit if my stomach beckons my attention. But perhaps because I am so interested in the life beyond immediate workings of my own body that hunger rarely surfaces to distract me. I really find that I focus better and am much more productive by postponing my main meal until evening.

On my one-day-a-week fast, by late afternoon, I am definitely hungry! The abstinence actually makes me fill my hunger with other things, like watching a sunset or practicing my yoga. I satiate my senses other than taste. Strange, you might say, but I find it a rewarding reminder of the many, many ways that I can nourish myself. This focus upon nourishing my life puts CR into perspective, and yet CR has been the main avenue for developing this attitude—go figure!

HARRY

I'm on a fairly severe version of the Longevity Diet, but I eat so many vegetables and other high-volume, low-calorie foods that my stomach feels pretty full most of the time. If the hunger is "there," I don't notice it! I am fortunate that the Longevity Diet is truly effortless for me.

NATALIE

My secret is tea. I have been on the CR longevity diet for over five years. At times it's seemed effortless, other times, a challenge. The excitement of doing something that was improving my health so immensely was enough to forestall any hunger issues. But after a couple years I started to have "Difficult CR Days." Maybe I was just pushing my CR too hard, but there were times when it felt very difficult. My stomach was just empty, and seemed to "demand" to be filled.

That's where tea came in. I discovered that drinking green tea filled my stomach in a more effective way than water did, even when I didn't add any milk or honey or anything else with calories in it. When I'm hungry but my next meal is an hour or two away, a cup of warm green tea helps me feel satiated. My CR routine is now something I know I'll be able to stick with for a lifetime.

Obstacles and Challenges to the Longevity Diet

We understand that one's relationship to food carries with it so many other issues that "just" eating less is of course not so easy for certain people. Aside from those who have a genetic predisposition toward overeating, many others grew up in families where food was used as part of a subtle, and in some cases extremely cruel, punishment-and-reward system. For these people, eating less can of course be a tremendous struggle. But it is important to separate as much as you can the actual nutritional purpose of food from whatever else you might feel about eating. If you are feeling blue because you've broken up with a lover, devouring an entire pint of ice cream in one sitting and then feeling guilty about it will not reunite the two of you. If you have just received a raise, you can find many other ways to celebrate than by going out for a lavish dinner. For any diet to work, you need to be aware of what kinds of issues trigger your food-related temptations, and break the pattern of emotional hunger by the deliberate substitution of something that will not "punish" or "reward" you with unnecessary calories.

Some Possible Side Effects

Assuming your health-care practitioner has given you the go-ahead to begin the Longevity Diet, you may do so with little concern for side effects. There are only a few that we can think of, common to only the rigorous versions of the Longevity Diet.

One is that your body temperature will probably be a bit lower. This might best be understood as a consequence of the body's increased efficiency; *it is a healthy condition.* You may or may not even notice the difference in your everyday life . . . though, if you live in a very warm part of the world, it might even be a big plus!

Another "downside" for some people: if your baseline weight prior to your switch to an extreme form of CR is already relatively low, reducing your calories may result in extreme skinniness! If you don't like the way you look when you're so much thinner, then extreme CR might not be for you.

3

ABCs of Nutrition

Even if you are thinking that the Longevity Diet is perhaps not right for you, please keep reading: This chapter contains information that *everyone* should know. It provides an easy-to-follow overview of the basics of human nutrition. This is important background information not just for those who will be following the Longevity Diet, but for anyone who wishes to have a better understanding of how foods interact with the human body.

The Key to Weight Loss

Nothing is more frustrating than the endless, intricate, ever-changing flood of nutritional advice that streams past us in waves far too fast even to dream of being able to catch.

The August 2004 issue of *National Geographic* tried to cut through this miasma of confusion over diet and health. The cover story was actually not about CR; rather, about the more general phenomenon of obesity in the United States. The goal of losing weight is of course related to the goals of the Longevity Diet program. However, the article is written from a different perspective than our last chapter: its concerns about what has been called an obesity epidemic center upon getting you *away from* the most unhealthful end of the spectrum of caloric intake. There is a presumption that any benefits aside from weight loss will just fall into place, as long as you cease your intake of fatty (or carbs-laden), high-calorie foods. The Longevity Diet, in contrast, focuses on moving you *toward* the most healthful end, concentrating far more positively on trying to optimize your health, and not just trying to avoid the diseases of obesity.

The magazine article poses the question of why we're so fat. And then—one can almost hear a drum roll as one begins reading further—the answer to this seemingly mysterious problem is announced: "Because we eat a lot." It's that simple—whether your caloric intake is 5,000 calories/day or 3,500 calories/day, the culprit is not evil fast-food corporations, it's not your television set, it's not carbs. It's you. YOU ARE EATING TOO MUCH.

That might seem like bad news, but it's not. It's *great* news. Because the solution is just as simple: You just have to eat less.

We urge you to ignore those diet gurus who claim the consumption of huge amounts of protein or fat will magically trick your body into "thinking" it doesn't need more food. Indeed, recent research is showing that diets such as the Atkins diet are not at all effective in maintaining weight loss. As Dr. Ernst Schaefer of Tufts University, one of the researchers now investigating the claims of these diet gurus, recently put it, "despite all the controversy about diet . . . a calorie is a calorie is a calorie."[1]

Just eat less . . . and eat real food.

What Is Real Food?

Healthier eating isn't simply about consuming *less food,* it's about consuming *fewer empty calories.* This is the key to the Longevity

Diet. If your diet currently consists of, let's say, 4,000 calories/day of potato chips, bacon, and beer, making the change to 2,000 calories/day of potato chips, bacon, and beer will certainly make you lose weight, and *certain* aspects of your health may well improve, but the bottom line is that such a diet is not CR, it's merely FR—food reduction. You are lessening your intake of what your body doesn't need, true, but without the necessary step of substituting the nutrients your body—in part via hunger—signals that it craves. This is why so many other diets fail; your body feels hungry because it is experiencing a "true" need: a need for real food. In extreme forms, dietary restriction characterized by unhealthy obsessions about food can result in **bulimia** and/or **anorexia nervosa,** wherein you deny your body the fuel essential for it to function. A nutrient-empty FR diet definitely sabotages your health and longevity!

TABLE 3.1

THE LONGEVITY DIET VS. ANOREXIA	
LONGEVITY DIET	ANOREXIA
The goal is health	*The goal is denial*
Someone on the Longevity Diet is motivated by the desire to have a long, healthy life. People on the Longevity Diet want to be around for a while to come! They want to be *present!*	Anorectics often describe their motivation as, "I want to control my diet, my health, my life," while the subconscious reality may be one of worthlessness. Hence the internal dialogue: "I want to be less 'present,' less 'visible.'" They often view their body as being larger than it is, and work to achieve as skeletal an appearance as possible. Often, they don't realize until it's too late that such a regimen can be fatal—that rather than controlling their life, they are virtually eliminating it.

LONGEVITY DIET	ANOREXIA
A scientific, practical orientation toward life	*A dogmatic, Good vs. Evil approach to life*
Because the goal is health, those on the Longevity Diet tend to keep close tabs on discoveries in nutrition and medical research, and are always "tweaking" their own diets. The vast majority would give up the diet if the same effects could be obtained with a pill!	The anorectic believes that food is Evil, and that corporeal flesh is Evil. Thinness is Good. And the more thin the Better. That's it. This Good vs. Evil orientation literally consumes the anorectic's life. Research about a healthy means of achieving weight loss is utterly irrelevant to the anorectic, who is focused on the goal of not having a body, healthy or otherwise. (This is why anorectics are not cured by a nutritionist, but rather by a psychologist.)
The Longevity Diet means good nutrition	*Anorexia—"FR"—means bad nutrition*
If the goal is to reduce caloric intake, other important parts of the diet—such as vitamins and minerals—cannot also be reduced at the same time. This is why we call it the "Longevity Diet," and why others call it "CRON" (Calorie Restriction with Optimal Nutrition), or, with a bit less hubris, "CREN" (Calorie Restriction with Excellent Nutrition), or even "CRAN" (Calorie Restriction with Adequate Nutrition). A proper longevity-enhancing diet regimen includes a range of highly nutritious foods that in many cases, such as green leafy vegetables, may be consumed without worrying about exceeding one's projected caloric intake for the day, since the stomach quite simply isn't large enough to permit this!	Anorectics practice "FR": Food Restriction: eating as little as possible, of anything. In a bulimic anorectic, this takes the form of overeating but then removing food from the body, via self-induced vomiting or purgatives, as quickly as it is consumed, before its nutrients can be properly digested. The result of either regimen is extreme malnutrition, in which the body's cells and organs are starved of the nutrients needed to function and rebuild.

Three meals a day of junk food can easily top out at 4,000 calories or more per day. And yet such meals usually constitute a kind
of overfed form of malnutrition: a diet rich in fat, protein, salt,
and sugar, but containing few vitamins and minerals. On the
other hand, if you eat three meals of foods with fewer calories—
whole-grain cereal for breakfast, lunches and dinners featuring a
range of vegetables, plus snacks consisting mostly of fruit—your
caloric total will be much lower, while your intake of vitamins and
minerals and other essential nutrients will be much, much higher.
Besides such low-calorie meals being aesthetically satisfying
(we've come a long way from the "mystery [fake] meat" health
foods you may have encountered in years past), most low-calorie
foods are low on the glycemic index, meaning they'll digest
slowly: you'll sustain your energy levels a lot longer than if you
just grab a can of soda and some chocolate.

To put it simply, the Longevity Diet, especially in its milder
variants, is based on *pure common sense!* If you're currently stuff-
ing yourself with junk, STOP. Stop believing those articles that
point out that this fast-food burger meal is healthier for you than
that one. They are *all* loaded with empty calories. Instead, select
nutrient-packed foods, and ideally as many fresh foods as you can.
More extreme versions of the Longevity Diet might require careful meal planning to be successful, to be sure you are consuming
the right proportions of all the necessary nutrients, but starting
out with a mild version of the Longevity Diet simply involves replacing empty-calorie processed foods with healthy ones that
have been prepackaged by nature to have their own panorama of
delicious flavors, often beautiful colors, and always lots of vitamins and minerals. Or, as your parents probably told you, *eat your
vegetables!*

What You Need to Know about Nutrition

Nutrition can be approached in many ways. If you want to educate yourself in depth about this subject, you may easily do so by enrolling in a nutrition program at your local college or by attending lectures at the community education wing of your local hospital, or simply by going to a medical library and reading about the chemistry of food. While much of what you learn might not be easy to put into practice in your own diet, the subject is fascinating, and the knowledge you gain will be rewarding in and of itself.

Meanwhile, here are some of the fundamental principles of nutrition that are essential for everyone to keep in mind when thinking about what to eat:

The Basics: Your Body's Essential Needs

Your body needs to get a certain amount of **protein, lipids, vitamins, minerals,** and, yes, **calories,** from the diet. Your body also needs a steady supply of two other items: oxygen and water. For the purposes of this book, we'll assume you know how to breathe and know that it's important to drink enough water (at least six glasses a day, which can include juices, teas, and broths). Let's take those other necessities from the top.

Protein

Protein is a general term for a whole class of molecules built up from smaller, nitrogen-rich chemical units known as **amino acids.** Amino acids link together to form all the proteins and protein complexes in your body. For example, the principal protein of your hair is keratin, while the principal protein of your skin is collagen. They are built up from different combinations of amino acids.

Your body puts proteins to use in a variety of ways. Protein is an essential component of tissues in your body, which are not static substances but need lifelong replenishment by means of additional protein. Another example of proteins are enzymes, molecules that control certain chemical reactions in your body by speeding up those responses that need speeding up, and slowing down others. Protein is also found in hormones, and can be used as a source of energy (calories).

Fortunately, we do not need to eat keratin to get the protein we need for our hair, nor collagen to get what we need for our skin. Whatever proteins we eat—be they from animal products in the form of meat, poultry, fish, eggs, or dairy products; or from grains, legumes, vegetables, or nuts—are broken down by our digestive system (specifically, by pancreatic enzymes) into their component amino acids. The body then uses the amino acids it gets from these ingested proteins, along with the other amino acids the body can produce itself, to construct whichever proteins it requires.

In humans, twenty kinds of amino acid are used to build proteins. Your body can actually synthesize most of them itself, but adults need to obtain eight amino acids from dietary sources. These eight are called "essential amino acids," since it is essential that we include them in our diet.

ESSENTIAL AMINO ACIDS

isoleucine
leucine
lysine
methionine (and/or cysteine)
phenylalanine (and/or tyrosine)
threonine
tryptophan
valine

For people living in Western cultures, the risk of not getting enough of these eight amino acids is very, very low. The main exception is the careless, so-called junk-food vegetarian who, by eating a lot of say, potato chips, may have slight shortages of a few key amino acids. Another exception might be a person who, due to food allergies, lacks the enzyme to digest a particular food source of protein, for example, someone who cannot digest the casein in milk, or a celiac child who cannot digest gluten. Otherwise, the risk is rather that you're getting too *much* protein.

Take a look at table 3.2.

TABLE 3.2

PROTEIN NEEDS

Average man	Average woman
65 g protein/day	55 g protein/day

If you want to keep it *really* simple, table 3.2 is *all* you have to think about. If you're a man, make sure you get at least 65 grams (about 2 ½ ounces) of protein each day; if you're a woman, 55 grams (about 2 ounces). If you eat a varied diet, as you should, you don't need to worry about whether you're getting the exact number of grams of tryptophan, leucine, and the other six essential amino acids that your body needs. Just think about your total grams of protein per day.

If you want a more exact formula for your daily requirement of protein based upon your body weight, use the following formula: 0.8 g protein per kilogram of body weight per day (or 0.36 g per pound of body weight per day—some experts suggest going a tiny bit higher: 0.4 g per pound of body weight per day). As your doctor will tell you, this may need to be adjusted slightly upward if you exercise a lot. A person who weighs 75 kilograms (165 pounds), will need around 60 grams of protein each day, if you're an average, healthy adult who is as physically active as most people are (and not pregnant or nursing). But, again, this amount of protein is so easy for the average person in the industrialized world to consume that you really don't need to worry about it, especially if you follow the Basic Guidelines at the end of this chapter.

TABLE 3.3

BODY WEIGHT (POUNDS)	PROTEIN/DAY (GRAMS)
100	40
110	44
120	48
130	52
140	56
150	60
160	64
170	68
180	72
190	76
200	80
210	84
220	88
230	92
240	96
250	100

Some of you may have heard about there being different "qualities" of protein. For example, the protein in eggs is often considered the "best" kind (actually, the protein in human breast milk, not surprisingly, is even better, but you won't find it on supermarket shelves). All this means is that eggs contain nearly the exact ratios of essential amino acids that people need. But we don't need to consume precisely the right ratio of amino acids in each individual food item we eat. As long as we get the amino acids we need over the course of a meal, we'll be fine. Indeed, many nutritionists now say that getting the needed amino acids over the course of a whole day is sufficient.

Lipids

Fats have gotten a bad rap for many, many years, or, we should say, *had* gotten a bad rap. Over the last few years, some authors of diet books, such as Dr. Atkins, have gone in the opposite direction, claiming that a lot of fat (and a lot of protein) in the diet can ultimately be healthful. But one point on which all nutritionists would agree is that if we completely eliminated certain types of fats from our diet, we would die. In Western society, it is extremely difficult *not* to consume at least *some* fats, so there is little danger of your not having enough of them. Indeed, advocates of high-fat, high-protein diets notwithstanding, most of us probably consume *too much* fat. Fat tastes and feels good, adding to the "richness" of food; it is no coincidence that we tend to associate low-fat versions of normally high-fat foods—low-fat cottage cheese, low-fat milk, etc.—with feelings of deprivation. As with protein, Western diners do not seem (or want) to believe that a little truly goes a long way.

The fat situation is a bit trickier than that of protein, however. In the case of protein, if you're an average adult in the United

States, Canada, Australia, New Zealand, Western Europe, or Japan, you almost certainly don't have to worry about suffering from protein malnutrition (known as *kwashiorkor*). But, in the case of dietary fat, most people in the West may well need to think more carefully about the *balance* of different types of fats in their diets. Danish physicians noted in the 1970s that natives of Greenland who ate large quantities of fish and other seafood had an unusually low incidence of heart disease and arthritis. And, of course, these Greenlanders consumed essentially no corn oil, safflower oil, or other vegetable oils of the sort that one can scarcely avoid in the United States. This led to research that forced a major rewrite of nutrition textbooks' chapters on dietary fats: it's the *ratio* of the kinds of fatty acids that are found mostly in fish (though also in many nuts and seeds) to those found in most vegetable oils, which matters for health. And this ratio tends to be far too low in the West, especially in the United States.[2]

While you may need to think more about your fat consumption than you do about your protein consumption, any imbalances in your intake of dietary fats are, fortunately, very easy to correct.

What Are Fats?

What most of us call fats are referred to as lipids by nutritionists and others in the scientific community. Lipids include fatty acids, triglycerides, sterols, and waxes (though we don't eat a lot of wax!), as well as so-called compound lipids—lipids complexed with another kind of molecule—such as phospholipids and lipoproteins. Lipids are the primary component of cell walls, and are used to make sex hormones, several adrenal hormones, and most eicosanoids (small signaling molecules that help regulate basic bodily functions like blood pressure and inflammation; see page 56). Lipids are also found in abundance in the brain, especially as the covering, or "sheath," around nerve fibers.

Sterols are, technically speaking, a kind of alcohol containing a fused four-ring structure. Cholesterol and steroids, as the names suggest, are examples of sterols.

Fatty acids, on the other hand, are generally smaller molecules that usually consist simply of a chain of carbon atoms with a carboxylic acid group at the end. The chain of carbon atoms can be completed surrounded by ("saturated" with) hydrogen atoms, in which case it is a saturated fatty acid (SFA), surrounded by hydrogen atoms except for one "hole" or "unsaturated" spot, in which case it is a monounsaturated fatty acid (MUFA), or there can be more than one unsaturated spot, in which case the fatty acid is a polyunsaturated fatty acid (PUFA). (See figure 3.1.) A common saturated fatty acid is stearic acid, found in beef and many other foods. There is only one common dietary monounsaturated fatty acid, oleic acid, which is the primary constituent of olive oil and canola oil, and is present in high quantities in avocados and many nuts. There are many different polyunsaturated fatty acids. Arachidonic acid (AA), shown in figure 3.1, is found in meat, and eicosapentaenoic acid (EPA) is abundant in cold-water fish.

Triglycerides are esters of three (thus "tri") molecules of fatty acids linked with one molecule of glycerol, a syrupy alcohol that gives fat its greasiness. When we talk of body fat, it is triglycerides that we are speaking of, since this is the form that lipids take in our body when we put on the pounds. Most phospholipids are just like triglycerides, except there are only two fatty acids, and in place of the third fatty acid is a small group of atoms containing a phosphorous atom.

A balanced proportion and reasonable amount of lipids are necessary for the very structure of the body itself, such the walls of your trillions of cells, as well as for critical elements of the

FIGURE 3.1

STEARIC ACID

```
    H  H  H  H  H  H  H  H  H  H  H  H  H  H  H  H  H
    |  |  |  |  |  |  |  |  |  |  |  |  |  |  |  |  |
 H- C- C- C- C- C- C- C- C- C- C- C- C- C- C- C- C- C- COOH
    |  |  |  |  |  |  |  |  |  |  |  |  |  |  |  |  |
    H  H  H  H  H  H  H  H  H  H  H  H  H  H  H  H  H
```

OLEIC ACID

```
    H  H  H  H  H  H  H  H           H  H  H  H  H  H  H  H
    |  |  |  |  |  |  |  |           |  |  |  |  |  |  |  |
 H- C- C- C- C- C- C- C- C- C= C- C- C- C- C- C- C- C- C- COOH
    |  |  |  |  |  |  |  |  |  |  |  |  |  |  |  |  |  |
    H  H  H  H  H  H  H  H  H  H  H  H  H  H  H  H  H  H
```

ARACHIDONIC ACID (AA)

```
    H  H  H  H  H        H        H        H        H  H  H
    |  |  |  |  |        |        |        |        |  |  |
 H- C- C- C- C- C- C= C- C- C= C- C- C= C- C- C= C- C- C- C- COOH
    |  |  |  |  |  |  |  |  |  |  |  |  |  |  |  |  |  |  |
    H  H  H  H  H  H  H  H  H  H  H  H  H  H  H  H  H  H  H
```

EICOSAPENTAENOIC ACID (EPA)

```
    H  H        H        H        H        H        H  H  H
    |  |        |        |        |        |        |  |  |
 H- C- C- C= C- C- C= C- C- C= C- C- C= C- C- C= C- C- C- C- COOH
    |  |  |  |  |  |  |  |  |  |  |  |  |  |  |  |  |  |  |
    H  H  H  H  H  H  H  H  H  H  H  H  H  H  H  H  H  H  H
```

body's signaling system. In addition, lipids are terrific sources of energy, comparable to the petroleum-based oil or other substances burned to run machinery (how many calories a food has is an expression of how much fuel it can provide).

Omega-3 and Omega-6

After our whirlwind tour of the complex chemistry of lipids, the following will be reassuring: Every single lipid the body needs can be made by the body itself, with only two exceptions: n-3 and n-6 fatty acids, popularly known, respectively, as the omega-3 and omega-6 fatty acids. Two common variants of omega-3 are linolenic acid and eicosapentaenoic acid; two common omega-6 fatty acids are linoleic acid and arachidonic acid.

The omega fatty acids are essential to our body because of their use in the creation of hormonelike prostaglandins and leukotrienes. These substances are essentially produced in all cells, and, in contrast to most hormones, tend to act locally and have very short half-lives, sometimes as short as only a few minutes. They are involved in the regulation of blood pressure, inflammation, smooth muscle contraction, reproduction (including even the process of labor in pregnancy), and many other vital biological processes. Because there are twenty carbon atoms in the molecular backbone of these substances, they are often grouped together under the term *eicosanoids,* which literally means "things of which there are twenty (*eicosa*)." There are different classes of eicosanoids, such as one that regulates inflammation. To function properly, some eicosanoids need to be "oiled" with omega-3 fatty acids, and some require omega-6.

Note: The body cannot "interconvert" omega-3 and omega-6 fatty acids; that's why both are needed in the diet. If you look at figure 3.1, you'll see that arachidonic acid has its first double bond (represented by the two horizontal lines between the Cs, which represent carbon atoms) between the sixth and the seventh carbon atoms, counting from the left. The left end of the molecule is the "omega end" of the molecule; that's why it's called an "omega-6" fatty acid: its first double bond begins after the sixth atom from the omega end. EPA, on the other hand, has its first double bond between its third and fourth carbon atoms from the omega end. That's why it's called an omega-3 fatty acid.

Omega-3 and omega-6 are needed in very, very small amounts, and cases of deficiency leading to the death of healthy people are nearly nonexistent. Indeed, it is usually only when placed on completely artificial diets that entirely omit one or both of these two fatty acids that people can suffer from a deficiency, and even then it takes some time before any symptoms appear.

Beyond the exceedingly rare cases of genuine deficiency, there is an additional potential problem involving these essential fatty acids, and that arises because the functions of eicosanoids made from omega-3 fatty acids are often opposed to those of eicosanoids made from omega-6. Generally speaking, those derived from the omega-6 promote inflammation, cell growth, and blood clotting, whereas those derived from omega-3 tend to diminish these effects or even have the opposite effects. Maintaining the correct balance between the two types of fatty acids is crucial to good health.

The body has some control over how many eicosanoids of each type get produced, but its regulation of such production is strongly affected by the omega-6 to omega-3 ratio in our diet, increasingly so as we age. If we consume a lopsided ratio of omega-6 to omega-3 fatty acids, our body will have a lopsided balance of eicosanoids, and this can lead to problems. For example, because many types of arthritis often begin with an excessive inflammatory response, a high omega-6 to omega-3 ratio in the diet can lead to an increased risk of arthritis. Indeed, a low incidence of arthritis in Greenlanders' diets is one of the things observed by the Danish physicians who first got Western medicine thinking about dietary omega-6 to omega-3 ratios.

Because in industrialized countries, especially the United States, food production has changed in such a way that omega-6 fatty acids are abundant in the foods most widely available to us, we are at risk for an overproduction of those eicosanoids made from omega-6 fatty acids. Look at food labels and note how often you see "vegetable oil" listed. Most vegetable oils contain a huge quantity of omega-6 fatty acids—one that is (a) greater than our body even needs but also, more dangerously, (b) difficult for our typical diet to counterbalance with the appropriate quantity of omega-3.

However, balancing your omega-6 to omega-3 ratio is very easy, regardless of whether you decide to follow the Longevity Diet. Just eat less of those foods containing omega-6, and eat more of those containing omega-3 (see chapter 6). Omega-3 fish oil capsules are another simple means to introduce the fatty acid to your body, apart from diet, although it's so easy to get omega-3 from one's diet that there is little reason for the average, healthy person to resort to fish oil capsules.

There is one slight wrinkle to the omega fatty acid story that should be mentioned before proceeding. We mentioned above that there are "variants" of omega-3s, and "variants" of omega-6s, and that there are several dietary omega-3s that will fulfill the need for the eicosanoid produced from the omega-3 class of fatty acids; likewise for omega-6 fatty acids. Nevertheless, fatty acids that already have twenty carbon atoms in their "backbone" are one step closer to being converted to the biologically active eicosanoids than those that don't have twenty, since the latter first have to be "eicosanized"—i.e., made into the twenty-carbon-atom variant—before they can be turned into the biologically active regulating molecule. This, in fact, is the difference between the plant-based omega-3 and omega-6 fatty acids versus the animal-based ones: the PUFAs found in animals (and fish) tend to be of the twenty-carbon variety, those that are very readily converted to prostaglandins and other eicosanoids. This is partly why it is often recommended that therapeutic PUFA supplementation—for arthritis, Crohn's disease, bipolar disorder, and many other conditions for which omega-3s are often given as treatment—be in the form of fish oil, since it has lots of EPA, the omega-3 fatty acid that readily gets converted to the omega-3 eicosanoids.

But, we repeat, unless your health-care practitioner directs you to supplement your diet with fish oil capsules, going easy on common vegetable oils and occasionally eating the omega-3 foods listed in chapter 6 should suffice to keep your omega fatty acids in balance.

Saturated vs. Unsaturated Fats

Another worry about fat—at least if you're not on a rigorous version of the Longevity Diet—is whether you are consuming too much saturated fat and/or too much partially hydrogenated vegetable oil. Both, especially the latter, have been correlated with increased risk of cardiovascular disease. The saturated fat in our diets comes mostly from animal products. Partially hydrogenated vegetable oils (which contain the infamous trans-fatty acids, a form of fatty acid not often found in nature, but which is produced by the **hydrogenation,** or hardening, process, and is especially dangerous to your health) are found in many processed foods. Some of the worst culprits are supposed "low-fat" spreads and commercially prepared salad dressings (see table 3.4).

Another lipid common in the West, especially in southern Europe, is monounsaturated fat. Monounsaturated fats are liquid at room temperature—that is, they are oils. The most common example is the main fat in olive oil. These are thought to be an important factor in the reduced risk of cardiovascular disease in Mediterranean countries, and are an excellent means by which to raise your **HDL** levels. Another source of monounsaturated fat is avocados. Adding monounsaturated fat to your diet is not as big a concern if you're on a rigorous version of the Longevity Diet, since your cardiac risk profile will almost certainly be excellent. But if you do not follow a CR regimen, replacing saturated or partially hydrogenated fats with monounsaturated ones is a wise idea.

TABLE 3.4

HEALTHY ALTERNATIVES TO SATURATED FAT

SATURATED FAT	MONOUNSATURATED FAT
Butter on bread	Olive oil on bread
Brazil nuts, macadamia nuts	Almonds
Cheese dip	Avocado dip
Cream cheese (on a bagel, for example)	Hummus, lox
Typical commercial salad dressing	Simple homemade dressing with vinegar, olive oil, and spices

Micronutrients: Vitamins and Minerals

Vitamins and minerals are, together, generally referred to as "micronutrients" because most of them are needed in exceedingly small quantities. This is why many people are able to fulfill their daily need for them with a pill. Compared with this, the amount of protein you need every day, if you're an average-size adult, would be about the size of your thumb, while your daily requirement of the essential fatty acids would be a very small puddle in the palm of your hand. The amount of *certain* vitamins, like vitamin C, and *certain* minerals, like calcium, could rest with a generous margin on the tip of your pinkie. But some minerals would be nearly invisible specks. These latter are called "trace minerals," because we need them in only trace amounts.

One characteristic that marks vitamins and minerals as different from protein and fat is that they never are used as fuel. They play purely structural and/or functional roles in our body. One of the most important roles of calcium concerns bone and tooth formation and maintenance. And many minerals and vitamins are parts of enzymes, or are used as cofactors in enzymatic processes. Selenium, for example, influences the "p-450" enzymes that help the body expel chemical toxins.

Do you have to worry about getting too few or too many vitamins and minerals? Well, the picture here is not at all as simple as it is with protein and lipids. If you are a fairly typical adult, and eat a varied, non-high-fat (that is, not necessarily low-fat, but not really fatty) diet of mostly unprocessed foods, and are sure to include several servings (some experts say five, some say seven, some nine) of fruits and vegetables every day, both your macronutrient and your micronutrient intakes will probably be fine. But most people, especially most Americans, don't eat that way. Thus, the popularity of multivitamin and mineral supplements. These can be useful, but only up to a point. For one thing, they do not preclude eating sensibly; lab-produced vitamin compounds omit many other important food-derived nutrients. For example, if you don't like vegetables, a small capsule cannot possibly replace the fiber of dark, leafy greens. Even more important, however, is that there may well be nutrients the essentiality of which we aren't yet even aware! As it is, strictly essential or not, there are many nutrients that are, at a minimum, *beneficial*—for example, many of the hundreds of chemicals that give fruits and vegetables their varying colors, such as lutein, found in green bell peppers and other green vegetables, which protects against macular degeneration,[3] or lycopene, found in tomatoes and other red fruits and vegetables, which protects against several forms of cancer.[4] No pill can account for all the nutrients that science will later tell us are essential, nor those hundreds which we already know are useful.

WHAT'S A SERVING?

- 1 piece of fruit the size of an apple or orange
- ½ cup cut-up canned, frozen, or fresh fruits (in 100% juice) or vegetables
- ¼ cup dried fruit
- ¾ cup 100% fruit or vegetable juice
- 1 cup raw leafy greens
- 1 small potato
- ½ cup of cooked legumes (lentils, red beans, navy beans)
- 1 cup of ready-to-eat breakfast cereal
- ½ cup of cooked rice, pasta, or cereal
- a smallish bagel (i.e., about the size of a hockey puck, not the huge bagels that have become popular)
- 1 cup of yogurt or milk
- 1 ½ ounces of natural cheese
- 2 ounces of processed cheese
- 3 ounces cooked meat (about the size of a deck of cards)

Also, beware of the facile assumption that, if achieving the **RDA** (recommended daily allowance) of a micronutrient is good for you, taking megadoses is even better. It is indeed possible to overdose on vitamins and minerals; vitamin A, for example, while beneficial to skin and bones, can actually cause skin and bone disorders if taken in high doses. Likewise, a recently published meta-analysis conducted by researchers at the Johns Hopkins School of Medicine concluded that even supplemental vitamin E, long thought to be helpful in preventing cardiac problems, and "essentially safe even when taken at extremely high amounts," increases overall mortality.[5] Please consult your doctor before taking *any* high-dosage dietary supplement.

Whatever diet you choose to follow, tracking the nutrient content of your meals over the course of a few days with nutrition tables or even a computer program (see Resources), just to see whether you might be running short on certain vitamins and minerals, is probably a good idea, and can even be fun! See chapter 7 for more on how to do this.

Calories

Your body needs energy, measured in calories, to run . . . in fact, you burn calories even while you are completely relaxed and lying still. Without a minimum average calorie content in your diet every day, you would die.

Unlike the other essential nutrients, a calorie is not a particular molecule or group of molecules. This is because many different substances can be used as fuel. Two of the previously mentioned essential nutrients, protein and (some) lipids, for example, are excellent fuels. A calorie is therefore not a specific substance, rather a measurement of energy.

The dietary sources of calories are carbohydrates, lipids, protein, and alcohol.

Of those, certain things we eat can *only* be used as fuel. This category is carbohydrates. There are two principal groups of carbohydrates: sugars and starches. Starches are simply groups of sugars linked together into long chains. Starches are very readily broken down in the stomach to yield their component sugars. Some carbohydrates, however, cannot be broken down by the digestive tract to be used as energy; they are called **dietary fiber** (see page 65).

Carbohydrates in and of themselves cannot be considered essential nutrients, since their function—serving as an energy source—can be filled by other macronutrients. But a diet where

all the energy came from fat and protein (or, for that matter, alcohol, which is not a carbohydrate, though can be used as a
source of energy) would be literally heavy and not very healthy,
simply because it would be loaded with far too much fat and protein. Too much dietary fat—especially saturated fat—is of course
associated with increased risk of cardiovascular disease. But, as
indicated, too much protein can also pose a health risk: It puts a
strain on the kidneys, and can even cause urinary calcium excre-
tion, which could increase your risk of osteoporosis. We thus recommend that you be cautious with diets containing high levels
of fat or protein and, unless directed otherwise by your doctor,
try to meet a substantial amount of your energy needs with carbohydrates in the form of fruits and whole grains.

The Essentials

Essential Macronutrients

Protein (or amino acids), which is used in building and maintaining body tissues and bones; as enzymes and hormones;
and as fuel

Lipids, which are used in building functions, in signaling functions, and as fuel

Carbohydrates, which are used as fuel

Essential Micronutrients

Vitamins, which are complex molecules needed by the body in
various ways, often as "cofactors" used by enzymes to facil-
itate the enzymes' job

Minerals, which are inorganic substances used in building
functions and, like vitamins, are often cofactors or compo-

nents of enzymes. They can also have signaling functions, especially in nerve cells.

Dietary Plusses

Many different components of a healthy diet are regarded as beneficial, but not essential. Let us just consider two major categories: dietary fiber and phytochemicals.

Dietary Fiber

Dietary fiber is of great importance because of its role in disease prevention. We know that diets high in fiber reduce the risk of diverticulitis and certain types of cancer—above all cancer of the bowel—in humans, lower cholesterol levels, and improve sugar metabolism. And, of course, there's the uncomfortable, if not life-threatening condition of "irregularity," as laxative ads delicately put it. (The Irish physician, Denis Burkitt, who first discovered the importance of dietary fiber, noted: "The only reason you have a laxative industry is because you've taken fiber out of your diet.")

Fiber is often divided into two types: soluble and insoluble. (See table 3.5.) Soluble fiber is the kind thought to be best at lowering cholesterol levels, and insoluble fiber is thought to be best at improving bowel function and decreasing your risk for colon cancer. There are many different types of each kind of fiber. As with much in human nutrition, given how little we know about fiber to date, variety is the safest bet. You should try to consume at least 40 to 60 grams of fiber each day, split among whole grains (individual grains, such as barley or brown rice, as well as whole-meal breads, bran, and other high-fiber cereals), legumes (lentils, black beans, garbanzos), and high-pectin fruits (apples, pears, peaches, oranges) and vegetables (artichokes, shiitake mushrooms, broccoli).

TABLE 3.5

SOURCES OF SOLUBLE FIBER	SOURCES OF INSOLUBLE FIBER
Corn	Whole wheat
Pears	Brown rice
Apples	Other whole grain products
Prunes	Most vegetables
Nuts	Popcorn
Oat bran	
Dried beans and peas	
Carrots	
Sweet potatoes	
Citrus fruits	

(Note, many of those foods listed, for example, nuts, contain ample amounts of both types of fiber.)

Seaweed contains important nutrients and is spectacularly high in fiber, too.

Phytochemicals

The word *phytochemical* just means "plant chemical." Phytochemicals are the thousands of chemicals in plants that are thought to play a role in human health when they are ingested. They are also sometimes called "phytonutrients," especially where a health role for a phytochemical has been established. Many of these, such as the many different pigments found in richly colored plants, are antioxidants; whereas others have hormonelike properties.

Scientists have known for a very long time that fruits and vegetables are good for you: they contain many essential vitamins and minerals, and they also contain a lot of fiber. More recently, however, numerous other substances in plants have been identified that play a role in the body's defense against such diseases as cancer. We know we'll die fairly quickly if we don't get enough vitamin C or magnesium or protein. However, the situation is different with phytonutrients. It is now thought that anthocyanins, for example, which are abundant in blueberries, protect brain cells from age-related damage; and lycopene, which is found in such foods as tomato sauce, protects against cancer. Will we die if we don't consume these nutrients? Some people might, but we don't know yet. How much of these should we consume? We don't yet know that either. There are no immediate indications of phytonutrient deficiencies, as comparable to vitamin or mineral deficiencies, this is why such nutrients aren't yet considered essential. But the tomato you eat today might well prevent a carcinogenic molecule from being able to damage your DNA, damage that would otherwise have led to cancer a decade from now. It is of course exceedingly unlikely that one meal will have an effect on your health! But a lifetime of a phytochemical-rich diet will greatly improve your health, and reduce your risk of dying prematurely of cancer or heart disease. Green tea and a range of brightly colored vegetables (especially green, leafy ones, carrots, and beets) and fruits are excellent sources of phytochemicals.

Some Basic Guidelines

Reducing your calorie intake is easier than you might think, and its benefits are so powerful that any other non-CR diet that has been advocated for health will seem both ineffectual and needlessly persnickety, as Katherine Tallmadge, the author of a fine book called *Diet Simple,* has pointed out in a *Washington Post* article about the CR study being conducted at Washington University (WUSTL): "I believe that one of the real benefits of the

COOKED VEGETABLES AND NUTRIENT AVAILABILITY

Cooking breaks down the cell walls of plants, which makes some nutrients more available to you. This is particularly true in the case of many nutrients in carrots and tomatoes.

Yet heat, over time, also can destroy some of the nutrients in vegetables, especially vitamin C, certain B vitamins, and many phytonutrients.

What to do? A few simple guidelines:

- Steam vegetables until they have become slightly soft.
- A little bit of fat can aid in the absorption of fat-soluble nutrients, which are found in abundance in vegetables—but don't go overboard. If you will be eating nuts with dinner or within a few hours of dinner, or will be having a slice of avocado, a typical salad dressing on your salad, or a serving of fish, then you're getting plenty of fat to ensure the optimal absorption of the fat-soluble nutrients in your meal.
- Why not mix and match? Have *both* steamed and raw vegetables. If science discovers that a few key phytonutrients are far more susceptible to heat damage than we realized, you'll be covered!

low-calorie approach is that it places important emphasis on the central issue: reducing calories, rather than getting diverted into seemingly important, but in fact, peripheral matters, such as carbohydrate and fat counting."[6]

But if you decide not to try the Longevity Diet, read on. A few simple principles will suffice:

- Include as many unprocessed foods (whole-grain bread instead of white bread, corn instead of corn chips, etc.) as would be practical in your diet.
- Eat several servings (at least five, preferably more) of fruit and vegetables every day.
- Don't eat a lot of meat, particularly fatty meat.

- If you want to avoid meat altogether, make sure you get some legumes (pinto beans, navy beans, lentils, nuts, etc.) every day, as well as some grains (pasta, bread, rice, etc.).
- Get at least twenty minutes of aerobic exercise at least three times a week. *This is especially important if you're not going to go on the Longevity Diet.*
- Check with a health-care professional before making *any* decisions about your diet or exercise regimen (including even the decision *not* to change anything). Get a few tests done, just to learn your baseline biomarkers. Having some data on a few basic parameters of health—for example, your cholesterol or fasting glucose levels—will be extraordinarily helpful to you in the future.

You may want to simplify things even further. Not everybody wants to devote a lot of thought to food or health, and we understand that. So, the short version of this advice to is make sure you eat a varied diet that includes less processed food and more fruits and vegetables, and try to run or swim or dance or play tennis or football or soccer (or any other physical activity that will be pleasurable and yet raise a sweat) a few times a week. If you don't want to try the Longevity Diet now, please tuck this book away where you can find it, should you someday be more concerned about becoming more proactive about your health.

Your Calories, Your Life

The Traditional View of Calories

Calories are a much more controversial nutrient than the other principal essential nutrients in your diet. Scientists have long had a pretty clear idea of how much protein your body needs each day. This is the basis for the standards set by nutritionists and governmental health organizations. The case is the same with vitamins, minerals, and lipids. Such standards place particular stress upon the *minimum* you need of any nutrient for your body to function properly.

In contrast, we know that when you consume *fewer* calories than mainstream nutritionists think is optimal, your health actually *improves* (up to a point, of course). So why do most recommended calorie requirements remain so high?

One answer might be that nutritionists, governmental health agencies, and most physicians simply have not heard of CR. Moreover, many gerontology researchers are still unconvinced of the potential clinical application of CR despite such extraordinary results in laboratory studies of its effects upon animals, and growing evidence that we may expect no less spectacular results in humans.

But also, notions of the relationship between quantity of food consumed and health have been so deeply ingrained across the centuries that top-of-the-line modern CR researchers still have a hard time convincing even other scientists and doctors that eating a minimal diet may be healthy. On an evolutionary timescale, it has only been in the blink of an eye that CR studies have started, ever so slowly, to change people's mind. And this is because it has only been in the blink of an eye that food shortages have ceased to be a serious threat to the average citizen of Western countries. Although, most unfortunately, situations of starvation or malnutrition still exist in third-world nations, in industrialized areas of the world we no longer see calamities like the potato famines that swept Ireland during the mid-nineteenth century. And when was the last time you met someone with beriberi (a severe deficiency of vitamin B_1, often seen in diets that are heavily dependent upon rice), or rickets (of vitamin D, largely stamped out now by fortified dairy products), or scurvy (of vitamin C, which for centuries affected not only sailors but mainland dwellers who did not eat sufficient fruit and vegetables)? If anything, we are surrounded by an overabundance of food that, like the little cake in *Alice's Adventures in Wonderland,* ever beckons us with the temptation, "Eat me."

From the standpoint of traditional medicine, CR represents a radical departure downward from a norm that has existed in the West for centuries upon centuries: "The more the better!" "If there's food, eat! You never know when there might *not* be food around!" Your body has the ability to convert and store energy in the form of fat. This ability was crucial to the survival of your ancestors. In the wild, food availability varies, of course, wildly. Therefore we humans, along with the vast majority of life on the planet, have developed the ability to convert stored energy to useable fuel when external sources of energy cannot be found. That way, if there's a famine, you can live off the fat of your belly when you can't live off the fat of the land.

Having a lot of body fat has traditionally been a marker of success even in other animal species: Think about the science programs you've probably seen on TV, where the alpha male gorilla is leaning against the tree with his two or three female companions. Compared with these companions and the other male gorillas, he is fat. And yet the alpha male is not viewed as a failure, as one who "hasn't been able to keep off the pounds." On the contrary, any other gorilla just has to glance at him to know he is the alpha male. Enemies approaching from the distance spot him and think twice about attacking. It is understood even cross-species that you don't mess with the alpha male. Until very recently, "alpha humans" also tended to be large. Napoleon notwithstanding, many emperors and kings were enormous.

Right up through the nineteenth century, in not only third-world but Western cultures, plumpness was also considered a sign of a person's wealth and congeniality, even morality; it is no coincidence that our image of a beneficent Santa Claus is always of an exceptionally rotund man, whereas such evil figures as Satan, on the other hand, are always depicted as scrawny (though one would think, if food were so sinful, Satan would be first at the table . . .). In Victorian times, a common term for a vegetarian was a "crank." A commitment to such an alternative lifestyle was considered eccentric. Even gender enters into the equation: Throughout much of the twentieth century, many people thought there was something amusing or peculiar about a male who willingly made a meal of salad, considered a ladies' delicacy. It was *manly* to eat meat. And even our own twenty-first-century culture retains that phrase, a "meat and potatoes man," as one implying a fellow who is figuratively (and perhaps literally!) four-square and dependable. It is difficult for doctors and nutritionists to fight this kind of message that runs so deep in our collective history, even while in this last century it has become fashionable for *women* to be slender.

The association between rotundness and success has of course reversed over the last few generations, partly because of the wide availability of extremely cheap food; in our own culture, far too many people who don't have the income or time to prepare nutritious meals from scratch have become overweight or even obese due to a steady diet of fast foods and processed foods high in fat and carbohydrates. But the notion that a bit of pudge is healthy is still widespread, despite the utter absence of evidence for it.

Some people, for example, feel that they need "bodily reserves" in case they get cancer or some other wasting disease. There may, indeed, be some truth to the notion that with *certain* diseases, a bit of pudge might at least help you get through treatment, such as chemotherapy. But it would be far wiser to try not to get those diseases in the first place. The Longevity Diet is one of the best ways to ensure that your chances of becoming ill or dying prematurely are minimized.

The Genetic Factor

As humans and animals evolved through periods of want, the message to overeat became encoded into our very genes, as a safety net to ensure the continuation of our species. The body itself—some bodies more than others—seems ever to crave more calories than it needs. Your body doesn't immediately start crying out for more foods containing, say, vitamin B_{12} when you get less of the vitamin than its RDA; the effects of such deprivation can only be measured by a blood test, or by symptoms that develop over time. But calories are different: The body cries out for energy-rich food when even a few hours go by without a meal. Many interlinked though independently operating signaling systems control hunger. Emptiness of the digestive system and low blood sugar levels lead the hypothalamus in the brain to send "Eat!" messages that are far more internally insistent than the inviting message written on Alice's cake. It's difficult for nutritionists to ignore so powerful a physiological reaction when setting standards for caloric intake. To them, the fact that such a "symptom" exists means it must be responded to.

Table 4.1 contains the standard wisdom about caloric intake. For even reasonably active adults, these recommendations are extraordinarily high compared with the calorie intake of people on the Longevity Diet.

TABLE 4.1

Moderately active men of average size	Moderately active women of average size
2,500 calories/day	2,000 calories/day

Survival of the Fittest?

Exactly how did this internal calorie meter develop? For the answer to that, we must step into the footprints of our ancestors:

When food is plentiful, it would make sense for you and your "tribemates" to eat a lot, make a lot of babies, stay around long enough to teach your young how to survive and start making babies of their own, and then fade away. But when food is scarce, during a drought, or a hard winter, or a period of blight-induced famine, it would *not* make sense to make babies. It would make sense to wait until more food is available, and *then* make babies. Otherwise, precious resources are being used up in a venture that is itself going to demand even more resources than simple sustenance. And here is the key point: *It is critical that your body conserve its resources to survive the times that are tough.* You must be youthful enough, virile enough, and fertile enough to be able to have children and live long enough to rear them. This means, in essence, that the aging process has to slow down during a food shortage. Resources need to be shifted toward the survival of the individual, not toward reproduction (the survival of the species). When evolution was sculpting us, what would have been available during difficult times would have been small quantities of seeds, nuts, berries, vegetables, and the occasional very lean meat (*very* lean, since the game available during a food shortage would itself have had slim pickings).

Evolution built into the genes of our most ancient ancestors a valuable tool for survival: When food is scarce, the body undergoes changes that permit it to survive, with all its vital functions intact, longer—much longer—than when it's "well fed" (in the old-fashioned sense). And there is considerable evidence to support this.

From an evolutionary standpoint, the Longevity Diet is about making your body "think" there's a shortage of food—how *much* of a shortage, is up to you! Think of the ability to trick your body in this way as a gift from your ancestors.

Your Body in Its Finest Form: Lean and Efficient

From a purely evolutionary standpoint, reducing your calorie intake will ensure you will last a long time. But what does this process look like from the standpoint of biology? What is happening at the level of hormones and cholesterol and DNA? While, of course, there is much more for researchers to understand about the biology of CR, we have learned a lot over even the last decade.

There are many theories of just what happens to our bodies as we age, and why it happens. Each deals with a different "system," so to speak: both the large-scale evolutionary systems just discussed, and systems as small as your enzymes, hormones, and the tiniest molecules within your cells. Each theory has predictions about what kind of changes we would expect to see if that theory is correct. Interestingly, animals on CR indicate the changes predicted by *all* the major theories of aging.

As noted, we do not yet have data on life expectancies for people following the CR regimen, because experiments in humans have only recently begun. But we have **life-span studies** from animals from widely different parts of the evolution tree showing that CR slows aging, and, in the short-term CR studies in humans, the biomarkers so far measured—such as fasting glucose levels, body temperature, and so on—match those observed in the long-term animal studies where greatly extended life spans were observed. Thus, it is very likely that the CR effect will be present in humans on the diet. Moreover, even if we can't yet prove that you can live to be 140 or more on CR, we *can* be certain that CR will reduce the probability that you will get many (if not all) diseases associated with aging, and that you will live longer than you would otherwise expect to on a non-CR regimen.

So goes the reasoning of more and more researchers who have been so impressed by the effects of CR upon animals that they have gone on the diet themselves. For example, a senior researcher at the U.S. National Institute of Aging, Mark P. Mattson, PhD, has placed himself on CR. So has James Greenberg, at the Health and Nutrition Sciences Department of Brooklyn College.

And Richard Weindruch, a student and former colleague of Roy Walford, has also tried the diet.

The Aging Process

Let us now turn to the various body systems and parameters that change as we age, as viewed through the lens of several common theories of aging. Interestingly, every one of these parameters is altered by CR.

These theories are of course by no means mutually exclusive. Indeed, each may capture a piece of the puzzle, or even be simply a different way of describing the same puzzle piece. Most of the controversy in the research community surrounds the question of which theory is fundamental, and which rather just describes a consequence of another theory. What is important to our discussion is that *none* of these theories has proved to be inconsistent with the biomarker changes seen so far in humans on CR. This provides yet more evidence that CR not only reduces disease risk in humans, it actually slows the aging process itself, just as it does in nonhuman species in which the antiaging effect of CR has been roundly tested.

We'll begin with the broad, evolution-based biological theories of aging.

Disposable Soma

The *disposable soma* theory of aging is, in essence, the technical name given to the evolutionary logic of the CR effect explained above. It is not so much about what is happening on a biological level when we age, as about *why* we age at all.

Soma means "body." The disposable soma theory holds that individual bodies are, well, disposable. What matters is reproduction of the species: individuals can be "disposed" of, so long as the species survives. This explains why signs of aging start to appear very rapidly once we are no longer able to reproduce.

If the disposable soma theory of aging is correct—and it almost certainly is—we would expect to see exactly what we see in laboratory animals on CR: during times of famine (artificially induced in the lab), the survival of the species is threatened, and thus individuals, or "somata," need to remain youthful enough to reproduce and care for their young once the famine is over.

Antagonistic Pleiotropy

Yes, that word is *antagonistic*: what this theory means is that the very genes that are beneficial to us early in life turn against us later on. *Pleiotropy* is the characteristic of having more than one effect, or one or more forms of expression. The immunological theory of aging (see next page) is actually just a concrete application of antagonistic pleiotropy. And the ability of cells to "commit suicide" to prevent runaway cell growth (cancer) early in life is the very same *inability* of cells to continue to survive and thrive much later in life. In other words, the genes leading to cell death are helpful to the individual when he or she is young, but less so as time passes. Even menopause has been theorized to be a consequence of antagonistic pleiotropy: depletion of the number of follicles in ovaries is thought to be important for the maintenance of regular cycles. Yet, in later decades, it leads to infertility.[1] More recently, CR research into the role of IGF-1 (insulin-like growth factor 1) and related signaling molecules has shown that antagonistic pleiotropy may be at play in factors that lead to growth early in life, but that accelerate aging later on. This particular antagonistic pleiotropy has even been called the "insulin/IGF-1 paradox."[2]

Antagonistic pleiotropy is of course related to the disposable soma theory, since genes that are useful for the species earlier in life become damaging to the individual (soma) later, once the individual has passed on her genes, and thus is, from the standpoint of the species, "disposable."

"System" Theories of Aging

System theories of aging look at the body as a system, that is, as a systematic whole. We will only mention a couple of them here.

Rate of Living

This is a theory that says if you live "faster," you'll die sooner or, as the proverb goes, "If you burn the candle at both ends, the candle won't last long." This theory makes intuitive sense, and has been around for a very, very long time in various forms.

The rate-of-living theory is also consistent with longevity studies in the laboratory and in short-term CR studies performed on humans. Animals and humans alike, on a CR diet, use their body's energy more efficiently. That means you buy more time. It's as if you have fifteen gallons of gasoline and you tune up your car so that it's running more effectively: the car with the tune-up will go farther.

However, there is an interesting twist here. CR actually seems to give the body more "living allotment." That is, it's not that the candle is simply burning more slowly, or only at one end. With CR, it begins to grow more wax. On CR, your body will use energy more effectively, your heart will beat more slowly, your body temperature will be a little bit lower. But also, the very amount of extra energy available to you will increase beyond merely the amount those markers of metabolic efficiency conserve.

Immunological

The *immunological theory* of aging was developed at UCLA by Professor Roy Walford. It is an example of antagonistic pleiotropy, mentioned above. According to this theory, your immune system, which is of course vital to your survival, starts to turn against you as you age. This can easily be observed in laboratory animals: **autoantibodies**, antibodies that attack parts of the body instead of defending it against germs, tend to multiply with age. These autoantibodies can easily be measured in humans. However, animals started on CR before they get too old stave off this rise in autoantibodies, and consequently live longer, healthier lives. Thus far, the CR effect upon autoantibodies has been firmly established in studies in animals, and will very likely be seen in humans as well.

Neuroendocrine

The *neuroendocrine system* is a complicated network of brain cells (neurons), hormones, and glands that govern, broadly speaking, **homeostasis:** the overall stability of the body's functions. A central component of the neuroendocrine system is the hypothalamus gland, located in the brain. The hypothalamus has a "master controller" function, monitoring and troubleshooting the state of the body. When the hypothalamus is working well, it reacts to the body's needs by changing the hormones it sends out into the bloodstream to deal with any problems.

The hypothalamus becomes increasingly damaged and dysfunctional as we age, as well as less in tune with its bodily environment. Once it is impaired, it regulates our hormone levels less and less effectively, which in turn damages the hypothalamus itself (above all, via excessive cortisol). Laboratory rodents on CR have youthful hormonal regulation much, much longer than normally fed laboratory animals. The evidence we have so far from the long-term nonhuman primate studies of CR shows the same changes seen in other laboratory animals.[3] Moreover, humans on short-term CR have so far shown the same preservation of overall endocrine function.[4]

Cellular Theories of Aging

Cellular theories focus, as the name suggests, on changes that occur with age at the cellular level. There has been considerable focus on these over the last few years, although the basic idea that when your cells age, you age, has been around for many decades.

Cellular Senescence

In 1961, at the Wistar Institute in Philadelphia, biologists Leonard Hayflick and Paul Moorhead observed that normal human cells only divide fifty or so times in a Petri dish. This limit is now known as the "Hayflick Limit." In the 1970s, a likely molecular basis for this limit was discovered: *telomeres*. Telomeres are "caps" at the end of DNA molecules that become shorter with each cell division. When a cell's telomeres reduce to a certain length, the cell stops dividing, and eventually dies. Interestingly, cancer cells (and a very few noncancerous human cells, such as germ cells) have an enzyme, *telomerase,* that puts a bit of the telomere back after each cell division, which is why cancer cells are essentially immortal.

Most of the cells in our body will not have divided fifty times by the time we die, even if we die in our nineties. While the Hayflick Limit cannot directly explain aging, just what role it does play is still being studied. It is conceivable that relatively short telomeres, even those long enough to permit additional cell divisions, are nonetheless deleterious in some way. Interestingly, recent research shows that lab animals on CR experience less telomere shortening than those in control groups.[5]

Wear and Tear

This is perhaps one of the most obvious theories of why we age and, in part because it's so obvious, it has been around for a while, indeed for centuries. The wear-and-tear theory says, in essence, that aging in organisms is a lot like the aging of inanimate objects: Like inanimate objects, living bodies wear out over time.

It is, however, a relatively weak theory, strangely enough. Despite its intuitive appeal, it can't account for why your body's response rate of self-repair decreases with age. Wear and tear is a side effect of life; aside from any external damage you might be aware of, your body is constantly repairing and replacing your tissues, cell walls, and DNA. This mechanism is not, in and of itself, aging. Indeed, it makes more sense to say that what *ages* you is the decrease, with time, of your body's natural ability to repair itself.

CR slows that decline in your body's response to general wear and tear, continuing its strengthening and revitalizing functions as it ages.

Glycemic

When it comes to calorie restriction, this is the most important theory of aging, since calorie restriction means energy reduction, and glucose is the most important source of energy for most of the cells in your body.

Glucose is a sugar that is ideal as a fuel source because it contains, in its very molecular structure, a lot of energy. Glucose is constantly present in our bloodstream, ready to be taken in as needed by cells all over the body.

It is in part because of its molecular structure that glucose can also cause collateral damage as it circulates around the body. According to the *glycemic theory of aging,* it is this damage caused by circulating glucose that leads to the pathological changes that occur as we age.

How can your body's primary fuel be bad? Too much of a good thing—any good thing—tends to be bad. The problem here lies in the ease with which the glucose molecule spontaneously binds to amino acids in proteins, changing the structure and function of the proteins. These *advanced glycation end-products (AGEs)* are thought to be responsible for most of the symptoms seen in diabetes, and, according to the glycemic theory of aging, for at least some of the changes in the body as it ages.

We know that CR lowers average levels of circulating glucose. CR may therefore slow aging simply by retarding the damage caused by excessive blood glucose levels.

Let's take a brief look at what happens to the glucose levels in your blood when you eat a meal. First, glucose levels rise. They rise faster and higher if you've eaten a **high-GI** meal but, even when eating a low-GI meal, glucose levels will rise. In response to this, the pancreas releases insulin. The job of insulin is to allow your cells to utilize the glucose for energy (though some cells, such as brain and liver cells, do not need insulin to use glucose). Some of the glucose is immediately used as fuel, and some is conserved for later use, either as glycogen (which is stored in the liver) or as fat (which is stored, well, you know where!). Slowly, glucose levels in the blood decrease, until you eat your next meal, and the cycle starts over again.

The glycemic index has increasingly drawn attention from the medical community because of its relevance in the prevention of type 2 diabetes. Most physicians now recommend that you select your foods with care to avoid causing a high "glucose spike," which taxes your pancreas, and, after time, can make your cells less sensitive to insulin, thus creating a downward spiral in which the pancreas is taxed even more, since more insulin is needed to do the same job, eventually leading to insulin resistance, and then type 2 diabetes. For most people, a sensible goal is to eat only small amounts of high-GI foods and to have a diet centered on low-GI foods, whose sugars burn slowly: a candle flame is all you need, not a blowtorch. This is why one often hears that "grazing" is better than eating just two or three huge meals every day.

Interestingly, a rigorous CR diet may make concerns with the GI of foods irrelevant. In CR studies in laboratory animals, neither different feeding schedules—eating twice a day, once a day, or, the ultimate in "nongrazing," every other day—nor variations in the GI values of foods used in the experiments, makes much of a difference in the resulting life-span extension.

In insulin resistance, the downward spiral of inefficient insulin has led to higher average levels of circulating glucose in the blood, since more is needed to achieve the same level of transport from the blood into cells. Basically, the collateral damage caused by all that glucose zipping around your body increases as the amount of glucose in your blood increases.

In a sense, the glycemic theory of aging could be seen as explaining both why people with insulin resistance and/or type 2 diabetes develop so many health problems and generally don't live very long, *and* why all people, not just those with type 2 diabetes, develop health problems as they age.[6]

Insulin and Aging

Interestingly, there is considerable evidence that insulin is itself central to the aging process. Indeed, studies of centenarians have shown that low average levels of circulating insulin are one of the very few things they all have in common.[7] This may at least in part be a different way of saying they have low average-circulating glucose levels—and these centenarians do indeed also have relatively low blood glucose levels—but it appears that insulin plays a role in aging that is independent of the role of glucose.

While much more research needs to be done, Cynthia Kenyon at the University of California–San Francisco, and Marc Tatar at Brown University, to name just a few of the researchers investigating insulin pathways, are starting to unravel the mysteries of the relationship between insulin and aging.[8] In the five years since the first edition of *The Longevity Diet* was written, many more details about insulin and related signal systems have been unlocked. We will address some of these new findings at the end of this chapter.

Whether or not insulin is fundamental in the aging process, or is merely a marker for some other fundamental process, we already know there is a correlation between lowered insulin levels and a reduced rate of aging. CR lowers circulating insulin levels in all creatures in which it's been tested, including humans.

Free Radical

If there's any theory of aging that you've heard about it's probably the *free radical* theory of aging. This has nothing to do with anarchistic political movements. **Free radicals** are, rather, highly reactive chemical fragments that can cause damage to vital molecules and tissues in your body. We need to go into some detail here, since this theory of aging is so often discussed, and, unfortunately, has so often been the basis of highly simplistic, deceptive ads for "miracle" cures.

To put it simply, a free radical is an atom or group of atoms with the wrong number of electrons. Free radicals *really want* to get the right number of electrons. You might remember something about "electron spin" from a high school or college chemistry class. Electrons with "up" spin need to pair with electrons with "down" spin for the molecule they orbit to become balanced.

Free radicals grab the nearest available electron they find, to get the right electron balance. There are two ways this can happen. One is that a free radical finds another free radical, and they share their electrons in a way that both become satisfied. This is how stable chemical bonds are formed. It is like playing dominoes: The basic technique places bars flat on the table end to end against each other, pairing quantities of dots, like with like. But the other way is that a free radical will steal an electron, which in turn creates another free radical: the molecule from which the electron was stolen. Once *that* molecule is a free radical, it might steal an electron from yet another molecule, in a crashing *domino effect* that can go on for quite some time. This latter process is a dangerous chain reaction of molecular malfunctions.

Free radicals also play a useful function, of course, such as in the destruction of bacteria by the immune system. But the body needs a way to arrest the activities of free radicals where they aren't needed. We have enzyme systems that can neutralize them very well. But also, antioxidants can neutralize (or actually "trap") free radicals. More about those in a moment.

Most of the damage done by free radicals can very quickly be repaired, but a little bit remains after each free radical "strike." The damage that even this small amount can do is known to play a role in a number of illnesses, especially cancer. Free radical damage to DNA molecules causes mutations, which can lead to out-of-control growth—cancer—of the kind of cell whose DNA was damaged.

It is also postulated that free radical damage causes the overall decline in body functions that leads to, or, rather simply *is*, aging.

Here, of course, is where the supplement industry has seen a golden opportunity.

The free radical theory of aging, at least in its broadest outlines, is legitimate and pretty straightforward: free radicals are "bad guys" that do bad things; if there were "good guys" to lasso and get rid of them, we wouldn't age as quickly. However, beware of the methods of over-the-counter antioxidant packagers, who are very sophisticated and slick . . . and simplistic, not unlike the snake-oil salesmen of yesteryear. In health food stores, for example, one brochure we've seen features a picture of a young woman's face, with a small part of her cheek expanded into a close-up view showing a few delicate-seeming collagen molecules and some small red circles representing free radicals. The red circles are little, fanged devil faces getting ready to chomp on the fragile molecules. Then there are some green circles with smiley faces, representing antioxidants. They are positioned to look as though they are guarding the woman's collagen against the devils. The next picture shows shiny new bottles of vitamins C and E (two vitamins that also happen to be antioxidants), whose manufacturer's icon—surprise!—bears a striking resemblance to an antioxidant smiley face.

What could be more compelling than such a simple view of health, one that matches our notions that the world is divided into Good and Evil, Virtue and Vice? Yet, for better or worse, the human body is not simple. The putative virtues of antioxidant supplements cannot make up for bad eating habits.

The fact is, *no* studies to date with antioxidant supplements of *any kind* have demonstrated a significant slowing of the aging process in laboratory animals. There do appear to be some health benefits to antioxidant supplementation, but so far, in the laboratory, the aging process per se has not been altered by supplemental antioxidants. Does this mean the free radical theory of aging is incorrect? Not at all! The more reasonable conclusion is that your body actually requires a certain level of free radicals—free radicals, after all, play an important physiological role, especially in the immune system. Thus the body may simply alter production of its own antioxidants to maintain the right balance of free radicals and antioxidants in the face of the onslaught of vitamin C or E that you're consuming in the form of a pill.

It has been known for some time that certain commonly consumed antioxidant supplements—vitamin C, vitamin E, and beta carotene—appear to have no health benefit in humans, and may even be slightly harmful to certain people, for example, smokers.[9] We don't know whether it is the antioxidant properties of these substances that are doing harm, or something else about them. More recent work, however, shows that it is likely that the antioxidant properties per se of vitamins C and E can be detrimental at least to one important aspect of health under certain circumstances. A widely cited study published in 2009 provided evidence for the *positive* role of oxidation in the reduction in risk of type 2 diabetes that occurs with sustained aerobic exercise. Exercisers who took 1,000 mg of vitamin C and 400 IUs of vitamin E did not experience this increase in insulin sensitivity. It is thought that the body's response to the increased generation of free radicals during exercise has a greater positive effect than the negative effect of the free radicals themselves. Vitamins C and E appeared to block the positive response to the free radicals by partially neutralizing them![10]

Unlike regimens that rely upon supplements, the Longevity Diet, via the shift in the use of resources required under conditions of reduced energy intake, actually lowers free radical production.

The fewer free radicals that exist in your body, the less your body will be damaged by instances of their domino effect. The result may be a longer life.

Miscellaneous Theories

There are many other theories of aging, some focusing on even smaller components of the body, such as the DNA inside your *mitochondria,* the small components of cells that produce energy. We find that CR in lab animals produces changes consistent with a slowing of the aging process as defined in these theories of aging as well. For example, CR greatly reduces the age-associated increase in damage to mitochondrial DNA.[11] Another DNA-related theory focuses on the decline with age of the organism's ability to regulate gene expression—CR also mitigates this decline.[12]

The fact that there are so many competing theories of aging makes it clear how far we have to go in understanding the aging process. But the facts that the effects of CR are consistent with *all* of these theories, and that all changes so far observed in humans on short-term CR are *also* consistent with these theories, strongly suggest that CR will greatly improve your health, and will most likely slow your rate of aging appreciably.

Update: New Data, Same Conclusion

Tremendous progress in the quest to understand CR and aging has been made on many fronts in the last few years. Many hundreds of new research papers have been published, several dozen on primate (both human and otherwise) CR alone. We cannot review all of the findings here. And we suspect that most of our readers are not interested in the niceties of the down-and-up regulation of various obscure enzymes and other molecules seen under conditions of CR.

What our readers have told us most interests them, and, indeed, what most interests us, are answers to three questions that can be posed in the light of new CR research findings, or new findings in the field of gerontology in general. (1) Is our belief that CR will work in humans now further confirmed, or is it called into question? (2) Does the research say anything new about *how* to practice CR? (More protein? Less protein? Fewer meals spaced farther part? More small meals?) (3) Does any new research into CR or the aging process suggest that some *other* method of slowing aging and improving health is available, or may soon be available—a method, even just swallowing the right pill, that might be easier for many of us than CR?

Let us look at the new research in the light of these questions.

Does CR Now Look Like a Riskier Gamble, or More of a Sure Bet?

As we pointed out earlier, the only way to be absolutely certain that CR slows aging in humans is to conduct a study that would last well over a century. We don't have time for that. Indeed, it's likely that no one ever will have time for such a study, which means that we will always have to look for other ways to assess the question of the applicability of CR to humans. We might, of course, discover a large group of genetically similar people who divided themselves into two groups over a century ago, the one group eating a conventional diet, the other eating a strict CR diet. Alas, no such group has been discovered in the last five years, and probably never will be. We continue to be impressed by the longevity of Okinawans, who tend to follow a mild version of CR compared with genetically similar "control groups" in the rest of

Japan, but increasing Westernization of the Okinawan diet makes Okinawans less and less suitable as an "accidental" CR experiment. (That Okinawans live longer despite the partial Westernization of their diet makes the CR effect of their early years even more impressive!)

What we do have now that we didn't have five years ago is more information about long-term CR in our evolutionary cousins, monkeys, and a great deal more information about short-term CR in humans.

Let's begin with the monkey studies. Three separate studies have been under way for twenty or so years now. Many new things have recently been discovered about the rhesus monkeys that are eating approximately 30 percent less than age-matched control animals. They are healthier and appear to be aging more slowly than their non-CR peers in every way measurable. The effects so far seen are precisely those one would expect if the results seen hundreds of times in rodent and other studies apply to species higher up on the evolutionary ladder. The regulation of glucose is dramatically better and more youthful in the CR animals, cholesterol levels are far healthier, and the normal decrease with age in levels of DHEA-S and melatonin (known to many as the "sleep hormone," though it also is associated with youth) is tempered, to mention just a few effects. In addition, CR in monkeys greatly attenuates the loss of muscle mass with age, a condition known as sarcopenia.[13] Moreover, the brains of the CR animals are healthier and have more gray matter than those of the controls.[14]

It's still too early to have the solid life-span data we have eagerly awaited. The design of one of the three monkey studies makes it difficult to interpret the existing mortality data. To name just one problem: There were only 8 CR monkeys, compared with 109 control animals.[15] We have more reliable data from a second study, although the numbers are still preliminary. Twenty years have now gone by since the CR study in nonhuman primates was started at the Wisconsin National Primate Research Center. In late 2009, the research team provided a lengthy update on the condition of the monkeys in the study. Beyond being healthier in all the ways predicted by the theory that the CR effect exists in animals that are very high up on the evolutionary ladder, we have some initial confirmation that these animals actually live longer on CR. None of them has yet broken the maximum life-span record for a rhesus monkey, which is forty years. But more of the CR monkeys are alive later than the control monkeys. Another astonishing finding is that around 70 percent of the CR animals in their early thirties (very old for a rhesus monkey) have no age-related diseases, whereas only 20 percent of the control animals are free of age-related diseases.[16] The older non-CR monkeys are decrepit and suffering, whereas the CR animals are generally healthy and thriving.

Not surprisingly, we have no mortality data from the human studies. Humans, no matter what we eat, live so long that it will be several decades before we have even tentative numbers on survival rates. But we do have many more details about the physiological changes that take place in humans on short- and medium-term CR.

There are currently two major human CR research projects. One is the NIA sponsored CALERIE study (Comprehensive Assessment of Long-Term Effects of Reducing Intake of Energy); the other is an examination of members of the CR Society International, which is being conducted at Washington University in St. Louis. Both are well-designed studies, though there are, of course, limitations to any real-world human CR study. The CALERIE study has so far been very short term, but the WUSTL study, which is looking at a large number of CR practitioners, some of whom have been on CR for many years, continues to yield fascinating and positive results.

The first dramatic report from the WUSTL study we mentioned in chapter 2 has been followed by equally impressive results. In 2006, it was reported that an important aspect of heart health was preserved on CR. It has been known for some time that diastolic function declines with age in humans. The CR Society subjects, most of whom had been on CR for over six years—some considerably longer—had much more youthful hearts, as indicated by measures such as heart chamber elasticity and rate of flow of blood through the heart.[17] Another study looking at short-term CR and exercise in non-obese healthy men and women in their fifties, both regimens inducing the same amount of weight loss, showed similar results, proving that some of the benefits of CR take place relatively quickly. (Interestingly, the exercise-induced weight loss also improved diastolic function, but not as much as CR did.)[18] Another new finding is that a thyroid hormone, triiodothyronine (known as T_3) is reduced in humans on CR, just as it is in rodents and other animals on CR. This is an important finding, since T_3, via its reduction in metabolic rate and oxidative stress, may be a crucial factor in the CR effect. Other new findings include lowered oxidation of RNA and DNA,[19] and lowered systemic inflammation.[20]

Based on these new findings, we must strengthen our suggestion that CR is a dramatically effective way to improve your health, and is almost certainly capable of slowing human aging. Just how much CR can slow human aging remains to be seen. But even a few more years of youthful life would be worth it for most of us, especially if those years and all preceding years are healthy!

The "High-Low" Diet—Need We Say More?

We have presented the Longevity Diet as, in essence, one principle—a relatively simple, highly flexible principle at that, which can be boiled down to this: Eat fewer calories, but get enough of all other essential nutrients. Roy Walford at times called the diet the "High-Low" Diet: lots of nutrients but few calories. Like virtually all CR researchers over the decades, we regard "enough" to be simply what nutritionists generally agree are necessary levels of these micronutrients. Minor disagreements may exist among some researchers—60 mg of vitamin C a day, or 80 mg? or perhaps 90 mg?—but otherwise there is broad consensus among nutritionists on what levels of micronutrients are needed by adults. All other aspects of the diet we leave to you to mold around your schedule, your needs, and, of course, your taste! We have adopted this position based on numerous studies in laboratory animals showing that neither meal-timing nor variations in the composition of the CR diet—more or less fat, more or less protein, and so on—has any significant effect on longevity, provided one consumes sufficient essential nutrients. Our question now is whether or not anything in recent research would cause us to alter our view.

Our answer is a slightly qualified no. The people in the human studies ate very different types of foods and timed their meals very differently from one another, but all experienced tremendous health benefits, and all showed positive changes in biomarkers we believe to be measures of age or rate of aging. But there is one exception: those eating less protein had lower levels of insulin-like growth factor 1 (IGF-1). The question is whether lower levels of IGF-1 are important in the CR effect in humans.

IGF-1 is an anabolic hormone with many effects in the body. The amount of IGF-1 in the blood isn't the only determinant of the extent of IGF-1's effects. Other factors can bind to or otherwise limit IGF-1 signaling somewhat, which is why researchers often speak of the level of "IGF-1 signaling," not simply levels of IGF-1. Early in life, higher levels of IGF-1 signaling appear to be needed to promote growth. Later in life, at least in research animals, reduced levels seem to be associated with slowed aging. Numerous studies have shown that mutations that reduce IGF-1 signaling slow aging in laboratory animals.

Curiously, in nearly all human CR studies—the Biosphere study, the CALERIE studies, and most of the studies at WUSTL—IGF-1 levels were found not to be reduced. Yet in each of these studies, all the other biomarkers of health and age were shifted significantly in a positive direction. Most of the people in these studies were actually eating relatively high amounts of protein. Luigi Fontana has shown that IGF-1 levels are reduced in humans if they lower their protein intake. Indeed, simply switching some of the long-term CR practitioners from a diet of, on average, 1.67 grams of protein per kilogram of body weight (as it happens, much more protein than we recommended on pages 47–49 in the first edition of this book) to, on average, 0.95 grams of protein per kilogram of body weight (still a touch more than we recommend!), lowered IGF-1 levels in a mere three weeks by 25 percent, on average.[21]

What do we make of all this? The evidence is strong that IGF-1 signaling is central, though perhaps not primary, in the anti-aging effects of CR in laboratory animals (the worm *C. elegans*, fruit flies, and mice). Reducing IGF-1 signaling via genetic manipulation or other means increases life span in these organisms. Yet in humans, *all* the changes in biomarkers so far measured that are also seen in laboratory CR animals also take place on CR, except the change in IGF-1 signaling.

The picture gets even more complicated when we look at studies of long-lived humans and IGF-1 levels. As Stephen Spindler points out in his review of recent CR findings, many studies show that very long-lived humans have higher levels of IGF-1, and interventions that elevate IGF-1 levels improve cognition in the elderly who have experienced cognitive decline. Yet elevated levels of IGF-1 are also associated with increased risk of cancer.[22]

Our conclusion is that it is too early to recommend a CR program based on lowering IGF-1 (or IGF-1 signaling). Avoiding excessive protein intake is wise for other reasons (which is why the U.S. government does not recommend extremely high levels of protein intake).

In sum: Lower your caloric intake and follow government recommendations on essential nutrients other than calories.

Other Life-Extension News. . . .

Our third question was whether CR research, or any research involving the aging process, has produced a miracle pill that has the same results as CR, or better results! It appears we still have a long way to go, even longer than we thought when we wrote the first edition.

In 2005, we were excited about a substance in wine called **resveratrol.** Some initial studies showed that resveratrol could slow aging in worms and yeast.[23] But even then, in 2005, there were other studies that called the effect of resveratrol into question.[24] What we were hoping for was a study in normally fed mice—which are much closer to us genetically than worms and flies—that showed a life-span extension similar to that produced by CR. Unfortunately, the only life-span study in rodents we have is a study in which resveratrol improved the health of overweight mice eating a high-calorie diet. This is a useful finding, but doesn't provide evidence for an antiaging effect of resveratrol.[25] A more recent study showed many similar though not identical effects of resveratrol and CR in mice, though life-span data were not reported.[26] We suggest keeping an eye on resveratrol research; but for the time being, we have no reason to recommend it as an alternative to CR.

In 2009, it was reported that rapamycin, in use in humans for many years as an immunosuppressant drug, extended the life span of mice, even though treatment was begun relatively late in their lives.[27] Aside from the timing, disease patterns were similar between the experimental group and the control group, meaning that the drug wasn't simply preventing one or two diseases, but was slowing the very process of aging. This is an impressive finding. Because the drug is a strong immunosuppressant, we can most definitely not recommend that you try it for its antiaging effects. But research is currently under way to try to find out whether the immunosuppressant effect can be removed from rapamycin without removing its life-span–enhancing effect.

The magic pill some of us have been waiting for has not yet arrived, and is not right around the corner. But keep an eye on research on resveratrol, rapamycin, and related substances. Meanwhile: Follow the Longevity Diet, which is the best way science currently knows to keep us youthful and alive.

5
Your Life, Your Decision

We are constantly amazed at how many people we speak with get hung up on the question of whether the Longevity Diet "really works," given the lack of any present evidence of regimen-followers living a record-breaking number of years. True, we won't know with *absolute certainty* until after the year 2100 or so whether the Longevity Diet in humans genuinely slows the aging process itself as has been projected, if the studies that have recently commenced even continue that long. But while the gold standard of antiaging studies—which is to say, animals (human or otherwise) living past the age of the longest known member of his or her species—can't be achieved for another century or so, there is nonetheless overwhelming evidence that such a diet will indeed slow the aging process, and the facts are even more solid when it comes to the effect of the Longevity Diet on diseases associated with aging, such as type 2 diabetes and heart disease.

Imagine that no long-term, controlled study had ever been done specifically on the relation between smoking and health in humans. Imagine that we "only" have hundreds of studies showing that smoking shortens the lives of a wide variety of lab animals;

that we have short-term studies in humans showing that smoking increases plaque formation in blood vessels, damages tissue in the mouth, throat, and lungs, damages skin on the face, and in many other ways appears to be extremely deleterious to your health. In addition, imagine that we also have many theories about *how* smoking shortens the life of the animals in the lab studies: about the effects of carbon monoxide in their blood, and of the high temperature of the smoke upon their oral passages and respiratory system, and of tar in their lungs; and so on. Now imagine that we can actually measure increased carbon monoxide in humans who smoke, the effects of the high-temperature smoke on the tissue in their mouths and throats, the presence of tar and other chemicals in their lung tissue, etc. And that not only do we see the lab animals that are exposed to smoke over the course of a lifetime often coughing up disgusting black stuff from their lungs shortly before they are going to die; we see humans who smoke for many years coughing up disgusting black stuff from their lungs. Would it make sense to say, "Gee, I don't know whether I'm going to quit smoking. I need to wait until the long-term, carefully controlled studies with humans are completed." Of course it would not make sense! When it comes to your health, waiting for 99.5 percent certainty to go up to 99.9 percent would be silly.

But it would not be silly in the slightest to say that you don't want to quit smoking because you love smoking. That's an entirely different matter! Same thing with deciding that you don't want to give up your current eating habits.

You may decide you just don't want to change the way you eat. The pleasure of dining on rich, fatty foods, the intense pleasure of *excess,* is delightful, and may quite simply be something you do not want to give up. We're not on any kind of moralistic crusade against obesity. Indeed, there's far too much moralizing about food and weight as it is—food guilt has in and of itself become a huge problem in our society. We should not make people feel bad because of the way they choose to eat (and certainly not because of the way they look).

You should feel good about yourself, about whatever decisions you make in life. But if you have decided that living a long, youthful life is important to you, try the Longevity Diet!

Our only caveats: if you are pregnant or trying to become pregnant, are not yet fully grown, have a history of eating disorders, or have not been to a health-care professional about beginning this diet, do not proceed with the diet. But, even if you fit one of these special situations, please keep reading, as we still have much to say concerning basic nutrition and health.

If you are pregnant, or even thinking about getting pregnant, don't try the Longevity Diet.

- CR during pregnancy has not been studied extensively. Either way, CR during pregnancy is a risk—to mother and child—not worth taking. Given what we know about the evolutionary role of the CR effect, it would make sense that the Longevity Diet could also make it more difficult to get pregnant.

If you are not fully grown, don't try the Longevity Diet.

- When begun before the animals have physically matured, severe CR stunts the growth of laboratory animals. Don't try the Longevity Diet if you're not fully grown!

If you have a history of eating disorders, we would suggest avoiding the Longevity Diet.

- People with eating disorders, or those who have had an eating disorder, are severely at risk of slipping into another episode if they attempt this diet, because they have a predisposition toward an unhealthy body image and/or unhealthy obsessions about food. If you have or have had an eating disorder, you should not eat fewer calories than have been prescribed by your doctor.

> If you haven't spoken with a health-care professional, don't
> try the Longevity Diet—indeed, don't try any diet!
> - Talk with your doctor before making any
>   significant changes to your diet. Always! We
>   should all have good, long-term relationships
>   with our physicians. Your doctor knows you, your
>   medical needs, your habits, and so on.

If you want to start the Longevity Diet, and your doctor agrees it's a good idea, you will probably have a lot of questions about precisely *how* to put its principles into practice. Part 2 of this book will explain the various forms of the regimen.

Before we turn to part 2, however, there are still a few remaining technical matters that we need to address.

How Much to Reduce Your Intake of Calories

The concept of the Longevity Diet is simple: Reduce your caloric intake, while being certain not to fall short on essential vitamins and other nutrients, and your health will be greatly improved, and your body will almost certainly age more slowly.

But reduce *from* what level, and *to* what level? The question of your optimal CR energy intake is one of the trickiest in the application of CR to humans. There is at least as much art as science here. We will offer three different approaches: (1) "weight watching," (2) calorie counting, and (3) measuring health markers (which should to some degree be a part of any attempt to improve health).

Key to determining how much to restrict your energy intake is the notion of **set point.** Set point is, technically speaking, difficult to define, yet intuitively it makes a lot of sense: it is how much your body "wants" to weigh, the weight your body tends toward if you make no special effort to lose or gain weight. We all have met people who find it extremely difficult to lose weight. Even if they are moderately active, and if they eat what and when their body tells them to, and not more, they end up very heavy. Their body still seems to "defend" a higher weight than other bodies do. And then there are those extremely scrawny people who have to "remember to eat" to not become even scrawnier. The first kind of person is one with a high set point; the other, with a low set point.

Laboratory animals, of course, also have set points. One species of mouse known as the "ob/ob" mouse (yes, "ob" stands for obesity, and this mouse has two copies of this particular obesity gene) has an extraordinarily high set point. An ob/ob mouse is so fat it almost looks like a "mouse puddle"—a flattened, circular, fluid blob with a tail on one end and little ears and eyes on the other. These mice have *really* bad genes! On a very severe CR regimen, begun early in life, these mice still do not end up particularly scrawny, yet they live 40 to 50 percent longer on this regimen. They can't be taken to much more extreme levels of CR without endangering their health, even though they are not at all emaciated.

Remember, CR is not about trying to be thin. Weight loss is of course a side effect, but it is not the goal. The goal is putting your body into a state where its energy economy is altered such that maintenance and repair are prioritized. This state is achieved when the body is given less energy than it normally "wants," which will result in the body weighing less than it normally would "want" to weigh.

Technically, set point is often defined as what you weighed during relatively normal periods of your life in your mid to late twenties. If you were training for a marathon when you were

twenty-seven, ignore what you weighed then. If you had to gain
fifty pounds to play the part of Henry VIII in your local community
theater when you were twenty-nine, ignore what you weighed during that time. Just think of what your "normal weight" was during
your early adult years. That's your set point, at least as it is often
defined by scientists.

Where the art of set point comes in, is that many of us have to
make some adjustments to that scientific definition. If you were
always training for a marathon in your mid to late twenties, and,
especially, if you are significantly thinner than everyone in your
family, your set point is probably higher than what you weighed
during that period. Your body probably "wanted" to weigh more,
to receive more calories, than it did during that period, but wasn't
able to because of your training program. And, of course, you may
be above your set point for cultural, subcultural, or psychological
reasons. Set point, in so far as it is genetically determined, is not
likely to have changed in the course of one or two generations.
Yet in the United States, and increasingly, many other countries,
average weight has gone way, way up. Determining whether or
not your typical weight during your young adult years was the result of your genetic program or cultural influences can thus sometimes be a tricky matter. But once you've got a good idea what
your set point is, you'll be ready to start determining your Longevity Diet target weight.

The "Weight Watcher" Strategy

With the "weight watcher" strategy, you will plan to lower your
body weight by 10 to 25 percent, slowly, over the course of many
months, if not a year or two. Early studies of extreme CR initiated
in adulthood in laboratory animals did not lengthen life, and in
some cases even shortened it.[1] The adult body needs time to ad-

just, at least for more extreme versions of CR. We will explain more about the "caloric descent" in part 2.

If your set point is relatively high, you can probably aim for a 25 percent reduction in weight, perhaps even more, if you're very overweight to begin with. If your set point is very low, reducing your body weight by more than 10 percent could be risky, since there are health problems sometimes associated with extremely low body weight (more specifically, with a BMI below 14 or 15). Remember, of course, to talk with your health-care professional about any significant decisions you make about your health and to get a few basic tests of the state of your health done before changing your diet. Tests of your health, along with a basic checkup from your doctor make questions of set point and per- centage weight loss less important, especially if your goal is pri- marily simply to improve your health, as opposed to trying to live to be 120 or 130. See sidebar below for some tests you should take. Some of these, such as blood pressure and cholesterol levels, are very likely familiar to you. Others might seem a bit obscure, but your doctor can explain them to you.

Tests you can easily do at home
- Body weight (taken under same conditions each day; upon waking is best). Your weight will of course decrease on CR.
- Resting pulse (taken the same time each day, under the same conditions, preferably upon waking). Your resting pulse will almost certainly decrease on CR. Most people on long-term CR have resting pulses between 40 and 60.
- Body temperature (and save the thermometer, in case it is calibrated incorrectly). Your body temperature should decrease on CR. Most people on CR have a body temperature 1 to 2 degrees Fahrenheit below their pre-CR body temperature.

Relatively simple, generally cheap tests your health-care professional can order for you

- Fasting glucose. Your fasting glucose levels should decrease significantly on CR. Most people on CR have a fasting glucose level between 70 and 85 mg/dl.
- Lipids panel (includes total cholesterol, HDL, LDL, and triglycerides). On CR, total cholesterol, LDL, and triglycerides should decrease. HDL should increase.
- Blood pressure (ask for this at every doctor's appointment; also, ask for weight and temperature, for comparison with your own measurements). Both systolic and diastolic readings should decrease on CR. Most people on long-term CR have blood pressure between 95/55 and 110/70.

Slightly more expensive (listed roughly in order of importance)

- T_3. T_3 should decrease on CR. Most people on CR have values between 55 and 90 ng/dl.
- Fasting insulin. Fasting insulin decreases on CR. Fasting insulin is usually between 0.8 and 2.0 mIU/ml in long-term CR practitioners.

The Calorie Counter Strategy

Another approach is to focus more on how many calories you currently eat, instead of your weight. If you or your doctor thinks you may be overweight, then pick a reasonable target for reduction in calories. If you are in your fifties or sixties or older, reducing energy intake by more than 20 to 30 percent for the long haul is about as far as you should go, unless you're very overweight. But start slow! If you're forty, and currently eat around 3,000 calories/day, and if you simply replace high energy-dense foods with low energy-dense foods, you'll very likely naturally eat less than 3,000 calories/day, without making any conscious effort to eat less. And you'll lose weight. If you track what you eat, you'll probably see you're eating 2,500 or 2,600 calories/day. Stay at that level for a few months. Enjoy your new way of eating. Then check with your doctor, discuss your plan to go down to 2,300 or 2,400 calories/day, get a few simple tests of your health done, and proceed. If you feel good, aren't too hungry, and want to get even more CR benefits, check in again with your doctor after a few more months, get a few tests done, and discuss your plan to go further on your caloric descent, shooting maybe for 2,000 calories/day. As long as your health is being tracked by a doctor, and remains strong (and it will probably improve greatly), reducing your caloric intake to 2,000 will almost certainly improve your health further, and poses no risks.

The Health Marker Strategy

Some people have the time and money to get *lots* of tests done very frequently—once every two or three months. One of our friends on CR puts it this way:

> I don't really know what my set point is. I'm a 5'10", 37-year-old man who weighed around 170 pounds in my twenties, I have a somewhat thick bone structure, so I wasn't at all overweight at 170 pounds, I just had some "love handles." Two years ago when I decided to try the Longevity Diet I more or less guessed that ending up at 145–150 pounds would be a good "CR level" for me. I'm not even sure what reduction in calories that translates to. But I didn't care. I got my cholesterol levels and fasting glucose levels tested (both of which were not so great), and focused first on eating more healthy foods. It wasn't really consciously following CR or the Longevity Diet, I was just eating more "health food." I

naturally lost eight pounds very quickly. Then I got more tests done after around two months, and saw that my health had improved. I stuck with that approach for another few months, then started consciously eating less. I still wasn't counting calories, but I weighed myself a few times a week. I started to read food labels to make sure I was getting enough protein. I knew I was getting enough vitamin A and C because of all the veggies and fruit I was eating. Same thing with essential fatty acids. And I was almost certainly getting enough B vitamins, but I took a multivitamin pill just to be safe. After a while I had to have a few simple rules to keep my weight from going above 150, such as not eating after 9:00 p.m., and not snacking between lunch and dinner. It was hard at first, but I kept thinking about the lowered glucose levels in my blood, the lowered levels of free radical damage, DNA damage, etc. It made it fairly easy to think of the last few hours of the evening as nonsnacking hours. They were my "hours of freedom from free radicals." And I pop in to my doctor's to get tests done every 2–3 months. He says my health is excellent, so, even though I'm being kind of "loose" about my CR, it seems to be working extremely well. I may drop down a few more pounds, but I'm going to wait another year or so, just to make sure my current plan "sticks."

The Elderly and CR

Older souls may be wise and strong, but older bodies tend to be wizened and weakened. We know from animal studies that older animals often don't adapt well to extreme reductions in energy intake. There is of course evidence that those who are over sixty and obese will live longer if they lose weight, but if you're over sixty and not grossly overweight, you should be especially cautious with your Longevity Diet program. You have a huge amount to gain, maybe many extra decades, but don't risk that gain by rushing headlong into an extreme dietary change. Readers over sixty or so (this is a somewhat arbitrary cutoff point, since the relevant studies have not yet been done) should discuss this program thoroughly with their health-care professional, and proceed slowly.

PART 2

The Longevity Lifestyle

The Longevity Diet as a Way of Life

Ready — Set — Wait

Remember how, in school, you had to address five key points when writing a review or paper: who, what, when, where, how? Let's do the same thing here.

Who?

You, and the rapidly growing number of people who have decided that the Longevity Diet is the most sensible way to improve health and vitality. But primarily, and most important, *you*. As you begin to explore and design a healthier life, remember that it is you, yourself that you live with. While that may sound rather trite, the life you move toward should be filled with things *you* love. And this includes what you eat: Your dietary choices need to reflect the kinds of meals you want to sit down to, not a rigid regimen of foods you don't enjoy. Using our simple guidelines, you'll be able to tailor the Longevity Diet to suit your individual taste.

Remember, this is not a "Simon Says" diet. And that is a good thing! The probability of sticking with a cookie-cutter regimen of foods you don't like is low. Most dieters fall off the bandwagon of programs that require them to eat only specific foods or entirely shun others, or that impose upon them particular mealtimes regardless of how unnatural those may feel. Keep in mind that the Longevity Diet is, in fact, far more than just a diet. It is a lifestyle program that enables you to take control of your body's health and longevity.

What?

The Longevity Diet, of course!

The Longevity Diet is based on extensive research in a wide variety of disciplines, and is now gaining popularity among open-minded physicians, especially specialists in diabetes, Alzheimer's disease, autoimmune diseases such as lupus, and inflammatory diseases such as rheumatoid arthritis.

The Longevity Diet is often described by its practitioners as the "thinking person's" health program: You will learn about health, you will learn about food, and you will learn about yourself. This knowledge—or rather, this lifelong path of learning—will enable you to modify your regimen over the years, as new research results become available, and your body responds to the program. Flexibility is key to success.

When?

Why not start now? Animal studies have shown that the sooner a CR regimen is adopted, the greater the overall benefits, including an extended, vigorous life span. As Ashley Montagu (1905–1999), anthropologist and author of *On Being Human,* said, "The idea is to die young as late in life as possible." Sounds good to us.

And remember Dr. Walford's words: "It's a shame to die so young, because it takes so long to learn how to live." You have many, many years ahead, and potentially more youthful ones, if you start the Longevity Diet now.

Where?

Whether you eat at home, in restaurants, at the office, in social situations, or during travel, even to other cultures, you can adapt the Longevity Diet to wherever you are. The diet is easy to assimilate into everyday life and special occasions alike. And there are no absolutes, as with many other health programs; as noted in our introduction, the occasional "cheat" does not derail the regimen, provided you get back on track as soon as you can. Kim Sandstrom notes that "the times I eat off plan are actually more deliberate than a 'letting down of my guard,' and it is easy now, after a year and a half, to get back on the plan at the next meal."

The first CR Society Conference was held in Las Vegas in 2001. Who showed up? Finally fixing faces with names that we had seen on our e-mail lists and discussion forums, we realized that CR enthusiasts were an eager and motley group of all ages and professions who did not need to wait for a centuries-long human life-span study to believe in and begin a health-promoting diet that could potentially ensure a very long life. We had already come to know intimately such details as our complete blood counts, lipid profiles, and food preferences, as well as the effects of calorie restriction on our respective lifestyles. By way of introduction at the conference, we stated our name, age, and occupation, followed by—just for fun—what we each preferred to eat for breakfast. "Oatmeal with a few almonds" started off the rounds; "Grapefruit juice and coffee," said another participant. The variety continued, from egg-white omelets with rye toast and a side of applesauce; to kitchen-sink smoothies; to an oddly precise eight almonds, one brazil nut, three hazelnuts, and four to five macadamia nuts over low-fat cottage cheese.

> After a day of presentations on biology, nutrition, longevity, and CR strategies, we were hungry! With such a range of eating strategies, we had a hard time choosing a restaurant: one person was a vegetarian, another preferred raw food, one simply felt like having salmon. In the end, we proceeded to a typical Las Vegas buffet, thinking that there we would each find something that would suit us, and in a way we did—the salad-eaters gathered garnishes from other dishes; the protein-seekers managed with poached salmon. But those were slim pickings from the general fare, and we refrained from protesting to anyone but one another.
> In Las Vegas, arguably the adult entertainment capital of the Western world, we thus experienced firsthand the difficulties, even in the supposedly enlightened third millennium, of dining healthily in public. Obviously, the Longevity Diet message had yet to reach such restaurateurs . . . or their typical clientele. And so began our mission. Determined to wave the red flag and offer alternatives, we find now that current statistics on obesity, cancer, diabetes, and heart disease indicate that we didn't make quite enough noise back in 2001.

How?

Chapters 7 and 8 will spell out strategies to help you adjust your health habits and guide you through a gradual makeover. And it *should* be a gradual shift; we do not recommend the most extreme Longevity Diet regimen for beginners, even if losing a lot of weight is for you a significant goal. Here is your agenda, in brief: (a) Consult your health-care practitioner before you start. (b) Learn as much as you can about your own baseline biomarkers and nutrition before you make *any* changes to your diet. (c) Use the worksheets provided for you in chapter 8 to track your progress as you proceed with the diet. (d) Sign up with an online group for pointers (see Resources), so you will have a support system that you know is on a parallel track with you and will be in touch with CR followers if you have any dietary questions we haven't been able to answer in this book. And (e) Stay current on the latest research, via news media, the Internet, and your personal health community.

Remember, The Longevity Diet Works with *Your* Lifestyle

- You can mix and match what you eat—protein, carbohydrate, and fat ratios—as long as you consume a variety of vegetables on a regular basis and observe the nutritional guidelines recommended.
- You can mix and match how you schedule your meals. Depending on your lifestyle, you may prefer to eat your main meal in the morning, or perhaps at night. It is the total caloric content of what you consume across an entire day that counts. Variations in your caloric intake from day to day are okay, as long as the average daily caloric intake remains relatively stable.
- You can mix and match how many times per day you eat, according to your lifestyle and appetite: three regular-size meals a day, one large main meal, or grazing on small meals throughout the day.
- You will discover which foods best fill you up. Some find that protein and fats defer hunger. Others find that low energy-dense foods with a high water content satiate them. It's up to you how to balance each meal with your appetite and energy needs.

Q: But, What, Exactly, Should I Eat?

Focus first and foremost on vegetables and fruits. Think of them as a rainbow from which you will obtain a broad range of nutrients:

- **blue**—blueberries
- **purple**—red cabbage, kalamata and black olives, Concord grapes, currants, plums, blackberries, figs, eggplants

- **red**—beets, tomatoes (especially cooked tomatoes and tomato sauces), red peppers, red-skinned onions, apples, cherries, red grapes, watermelon, cranberries, strawberries, raspberries, pomegranates, rhubarb
- **orange**—carrots, winter squash, sweet potatoes, cantaloupe and other orange melons, oranges, clementines, tangerines, apricots, peaches, nectarines, mangoes, persimmons, papayas
- **yellow**—summer squash, corn, yellow-skinned onions, bananas, lemons, grapefruit, pineapple, star fruit
- **green**—especially cabbage and Chinese (napa) cabbage, romaine lettuce, bok choy, broccoli, Brussels sprouts, kale, collards, Swiss chard, spinach, beet greens, mustard greens, and turnip greens; but also asparagus, okra, cucumbers, zucchini, green onions and leeks, green peppers, celery, green olives, avocados, pears, green grapes, green apples, kiwis, honeydew and other green melons, limes (remember, wax or green beans and peas are actually legumes—and good for you, too)
- **white**—cauliflower, turnips, rutabagas, white potatoes, garlic, mushrooms, jicama, lychee

Although many phytonutrients have been synthesized and made available in supplement form, we do not recommend them: such supplements leave out important, if not essential, nutrients found only in genuine foods.

Plants won't be the *only* thing you'll be eating, but should and indeed shall form the "bulk" of your diet: Plants are low in calories so you can eat a lot of them, and they provide the fiber to keep your digestive system moving. They also have a low **energy density,** which means that their water and/or fiber content is high and hence they will satiate you more than the equivalent volume of most nonvegetable foods.

Vegetables can be enjoyed in many different ways—raw as finger foods (the only notable exceptions: potatoes, sweet potatoes, artichokes, okra, and Brussels sprouts), in soups or salads, extracted as juices, steamed, or stir-fried. Fruit can be eaten out of hand or in a salad, but also incorporated into gelled or baked desserts, drunk as juice or blended into smoothies, or frozen as sorbets and granitas. If you've always hated a particular vegetable or fruit when prepared a particular way, give it another chance in another form or two before rejecting it entirely—and, if you have never sampled some of the above foods at all, buy them in small quantities and experiment. Discover the heady delights of flavored mustards, nut oils, and herb- or fruit-steeped vinegars; stock your pantry with a variety of spices, low-fat dips, and light sauces. Read vegetarian and vegan cookbooks and magazines for inspiration—but if you like to eat meat, just lessen the quantity of it that you consume, while upping the vegetable count. For example, if you love old-fashioned chicken soup, prepare a potful with only one chicken breast and lots of root vegetables, rather than using a whole chicken plus only one carrot, celery rib, and onion. Substitute more flavorful, nutrient-rich fruits or vegetables than celery when preparing a poultry or fish salad (plain old tuna salad takes on a whole new dimension when paired with grated carrots, chopped red cabbage, chopped fresh cranberries or raspberries, or chopped apple and walnuts). See what happens if you mix various fruit juices with various flavors of soy milk (an amazing combination is mango juice mixed one part to two of chocolate-flavored soy). Play with your food!

When asked for advice on initiating a plant-based Longevity Diet, Dean suggested: "Buy one of everything in the produce aisle, and start chopping and chomping!"

Q: When Should I Eat?

Peter Voss, a CR practitioner of thirteen years, eats many small meals per day. Lisa does not eat until noon, when she will drink a glass of kefir or vegetable juice and have a light protein meal. Dean Pomerleau, a veteran in the CR Society, eats two square meals a day, in the morning and the evening, just as Brian does. And April Smith, a savvy thirty-five-year-old, eats differently every day.

Explore what the best time of day may be for you to eat a protein-rich meal. Some people on the Longevity Diet find that protein is what satiates them the most. If your stomach yells at you in the afternoon, it might make sense to have protein at noon. Or, if you refrain from eating after 7:00 p.m., a strategy adopted by some people on strict versions of the diet, then a high-protein breakfast may be an important meal for you.

Many studies show that most people will be more alert throughout the day if they've begun with a nutritious meal. But even though most nutrition and diet books insist that breakfast is the most important meal of the day, it might not work for you. So if you simply don't like breakfast, and you don't feel any worse for the wear without it, don't feel compelled to eat it. Or, if you simply can't face solids at that hour, a smoothie combining milk or soy milk, such fruit as bananas or blueberries, and a little flaxseed oil might be the perfect compromise.

Q: Wait: Won't I Be Hungry?

You may be hungry, at least at first. But we encourage you to experiment and learn which foods fill you up the most, what kinds of foods deter your hunger the most, and which of your hunger cues actually don't relate to food at all, but to particular settings or emotions. (Technically, these are, in fact, three separate issues.) Each of the major elements that make up foods—protein, fats, carbohydrates, fiber, sugar, and water—has a specific effect on satiety, both short-term (degree of fullness) and long-term (degree of hunger deterrence).

Let's place two meals side by side: One is piled high with a large assortment of vegetables, including spinach, broccoli, cabbage, red pepper, mushrooms, sweet potato, plus some cooked grains, a glass of milk, and a slender piece of meat. This meal is mostly vegetables with 3 ounces (20 grams chicken to 40 grams beef) of protein. It totals 650 calories and is roughly 28 percent protein, 49 percent carbohydrates, and 23 percent healthy fats.

The other meal includes a generous (3.5 ounce) piece of salmon, 1 tablespoon of olive oil–sautéed red pepper fajitas, broccoli, carrots, a sauce made of tomato paste and ricotta cheese, and a glass of milk. This meal totals 640 calories, but the protein and carbohydrate totals are 33 and 32 percent, respectively, while the fat content is 35 percent.

Which meal would you prefer? Nutritionally, they actually differ only slightly: The veggie-based meal is lower in cholesterol and sodium, and it is higher in fiber and has a much higher water content. The salmon and fajitas–based meal is higher in some vitamins. They are both healthy, nutritious meals. But which would fill you up the most?

The vegetable dish is based on one of Dr. Walford's classic salad recipes (see Dr. Walford's All-in-One Vegetable Salad). Vegetables have a high water content, plenty of fiber, and are low in calories, hence you can eat a lot of them. This meal will make you feel more immediately full. The fajitas, sautéed in heart-healthy olive oil, along with the additional omega-3 fatty acids in the salmon and the fat content of the ricotta cheese sauce, will take longer to digest, and this may sustain you through your hunger and your stomach through its fantasies. You see, both methods work, see which one works best for you!

Q. How Much Protein Should I Eat?

Some people following the Longevity Diet believe it is important to eat extra protein. There is actually little solid empirical evidence for this, but there are some theoretical reasons why this might be wise. Peter, for example, is especially careful to get lots of protein. According to U.S. government recommendations, he would only need 52 grams of protein for his current weight of 130 pounds. Yet, three years into his CR program, he actually increased his protein intake by 10 grams per day, from 75, already more than the government recommendations would indicate, to 85 grams. We don't yet know whether unusual increases in protein intake are indicated for most people on CR, but anyone on CR, especially very extreme CR, should, of course, be followed by a physician. Based on your exercise habits and other needs peculiar to your own life and body, you and your physician can determine a level of protein intake that makes sense for you.

Note, however, that during the weight loss phase of the diet, as opposed to the "maintenance phase," it might be important to get more protein than you otherwise might need. Whether you prefer fish, lean meats, poultry, legumes, or soy products, this is, fortunately, very easy to do!

If you are a vegetarian, low-fat dairy products, legumes, nuts, soy, and perhaps tempeh are already your primary protein sources. Include smaller amounts of grains, brown rice, quinoa, rye, wheat berries, and such whole cereals as amaranth, to build complementary protein sources. If you eat eggs, omelets made with more egg whites than yolks are an excellent source of protein, as are soufflés. These protein recommendations may seem difficult to attain if you are a vegan, that is, if you eat no animal products whatsoever, not even cheese or milk. Lisa was a vegan for six years. The combination, however, of low body fat, menopause, and having practiced calorie restriction for fifteen years primed her for weakening bones. Calcium is an essential nutrient that is difficult to get enough of if you avoid dairy products, even if you conscientiously eat bowls and bowls of green leafy vegetables and lots of tofu. Remember that porous bones are a possible side effect with long-term calorie restriction. So, if you chose to avoid dairy products, consider taking supplements. Lisa now includes kefir, yogurt, and cottage cheese in her diet.

Q. What Kind of Fats Should I Eat?

An oil is an oil when it comes to calories—100 percent fat. But when it comes to nutritional benefits, all oils are not equal. Consume predominantly monounsaturated fats, avoid saturated fats, and aim for more of the omega-3 form of polyunsaturated fats than the omega-6 form. Most oils consist almost entirely of these four types of fat, in different combinations. The most commonly available and healthy monounsaturated fats are olive and canola oils. Canola oil is preferable for baking, and is less expensive than olive oil; it also has more omega-3 than all other commonly available cooking oils. We prefer the taste, however, of olive oil in stir-fries. And there is nothing like the fragrance of a good olive oil in salads!

Evidence suggests that olive oil may protect against breast cancer.[1] A study conducted by the Harvard School of Public Health and the Athens School of Public Health on over 2,000 women indicated a 25 percent reduction in breast cancer for women who ate more than a single serving of olive oil a day. These study results were confirmed in 2008 by research at the Catalonian Institute of Oncology in Spain.[2] The bioactivity of polyphenols (natural antioxidants) found in olive oil are able to reduce tumors, and are being researched to develop more effective drugs to combat breast cancer. But remember, be moderate—even olive oil is still 100 percent fat.

Olive oils are pressed from the whole, ripe fruit of the olive, and are hence "fruit" oils, as compared to "seed oils," such as flax or walnut. *Virgin* olive oils are the only unrefined oil available to the mass market. By the time an oil is bleached, processed, and deodorized, it is robbed of its natural antioxidants, phytosterols (found in pigment), and other nutrients. *Pure* olive oils have been refined, despite the contradiction in the name! *Light* or *extra-light* olive oils refer to color and flavor, not calories! This olive oil is also refined, stripped of its olive taste and color. Avoid the refined oils, and select extra-virgin or virgin olive oil.

Olive oils are also classified by acidity, color, flavor, and aroma. Their taste varies according to the climate, soil, variety of tree, and ripeness of the fruit when picked. Similar to wine, the etiquette of the lofty olive, called "liquid gold" by Homer, has become quite sophisticated. Oils are graded according to their bitterness, whether they are pungent, fruity, musty, or oxidized (another term for a rancid flavor). *Consumer Reports* defines fruity as "a high-quality oil that may have the flavor and aroma of ripe olives—nutty, buttery, or floral. Or it can have a 'green olive' character, with flavors and aromas reminiscent of grass, vegetables, herbs, green banana, green apple, eucalyptus, or mint."[3]

Extra-virgin is the prima donna of olive oils. Generally used in smaller amounts on salads and pasta, a quality extra-virgin olive oil may cost more, but its robust flavor can virtually make the dish. Olive oils that are rich in color are generally more pungent, while the lighter varieties may be mild or even taste-free.

You may prefer a richer extra-virgin olive oil for salads, roasted vegetables, and pasta, but a milder, less expensive virgin olive oil for stir-fries and sautéing.

Flaxseed oil is the richest source of omega-3 fatty acids, among the vegetable oils. We always add a little flaxseed oil to salads. You may also grind flaxseed (available at health food stores) in a coffee grinder and add the ground seeds, rich with their freshly released oil, to your salad, smoothie, or vegetables. Take care never to heat flaxseed oil, though it may be sprinkled on cooked foods. This is the only oil that needs to be kept cool to remain fresh; find it in the refrigerator case at your health food store, and pop it into your fridge as soon as you bring it home.

Walnut and hemp oils are runners-up after olive, canola, and flaxseed oils. They contain a higher percentage of omega-6 fatty acid than the omega-3, but are still healthier than other mainstream fats and oils (butter, soy, safflower), and will offer variety to your meals. Hemp oil has a rich, lightly nutty taste that nicely complements a steamed vegetable salad.

Foods High in Omega-3
- Chinook salmon, halibut, scallops, sardines, herring (other fish from very cold waters)
- canola, olive, flaxseed, hemp, and walnut oils
- flaxseeds, walnuts
- kale, collard greens (other green leafy vegetables)
- soybeans, navy or kidney beans, tofu

Foods High in Omega-6
- corn, safflower, cottonseed, and sunflower oils

Energy Density

Energy density in food is a relative newcomer to many of us, familiar as we are with other measures of nutrition in food, such as RDAs, Daily Food Values, and percentage of calories from protein and fat. Many people on the Longevity Diet simply aim for foods that have high nutrient density. If you are trying to eat fewer calories (i.e., are trying to take in less energy), what matters most is that you get more nutrients *per calorie*; focusing on foods with high nutrient density is simply a way of achieving that goal.

Energy density is an entirely different measurement of food. And it isn't precisely the inverse of nutrient density. Around the turn of the twenty-first century, Barbara Rolls, PhD, along with her colleagues at Pennsylvania State University, studied the science of satiety: What makes us feel full when we eat? They compared foods that are high in fat and hence in calories with foods that are low-calorie but have a high water content. Water adds weight and volume to food without adding calories. In their research, subjects reported being satiated by fewer calories on the low energy-dense meals. The researchers drew several conclusions from this: People are sensitive to the volume consumed in the stomach, as well as to portion size.

Consider two plates with the same calorie content, one piled high with vegetables and a small portion of fish, the other with fish and French fries. The oils in the fish and chips meal have a high energy density, and the portion size will be much smaller for the same amount of calories. But the veggie and fish dish provides more nutrient diversity and a richer range of flavors.

Energy density concerns the amount of calories in a set measurement of a particular food versus the quantity you should reasonably eat of that food. For example, 1 ounce of grapes has 20 calories, whereas 1 ounce of raisins has 84. What is the difference? Again, water content matters. Foods that provide many calories in a small portion of food, like the raisins, are high energy-dense foods; foods that feature fewer calories for the same weight of food, the grapes, are low energy-dense. This dietary strategy is now recognized as Volumetrics.[4]

The water in foods is one of the ingredients that fills you up, as is fiber. Fiber lowers energy density by providing bulk, with few calories. Foods that have both water and fiber, such as fresh vegetables and fruit, soups, healthy cereals with milk, and smoothies, are both filling and, depending on the ingredients, low in calories. If you drink a glass of water before a meal, it will not be nearly as satisfying as when the water is incorporated into the meal, as with a soup. And when combined with fiber-rich foods, water dilutes the calories, and both the fiber and the water fill you up.

Nutrient Density

High nutrient-dense foods are healthy, nutritious foods, packed with vitamins, minerals, and other essential nutrients. Foods can be nutrient dense and be low in calories, or, surprisingly, nutrient dense and high in calories. The staples of the Longevity Diet are foods that are both nutrient dense and low in calories.

Energy Density

Low energy-dense foods are high in volume and low in calories. Since water has an energy density of zero, foods with a high water content are low energy-dense foods, and therefore high in volume. Eating these foods means you eat more food yet fewer calories. High energy density means that the energy in the food is dense, and thus smaller; less filling portions contain more calories.

To get the best of both worlds, we should try to eat nutrient-dense/low-calorie meals that are composed of low energy-dense foods. Now that is a tongue twister! But it's not that complicated: Choose foods that are high in essential nutrients but low in calories and high in volume (fiber, which is indigestible, or water), and you'll feel satiated yet won't have eaten a high-calorie meal. A few simple changes to your diet are a good way to start. For example, if you like pasta dishes, use whole-grain pasta instead of noodles made from bleached flour, and add lots of vegetables to the dish. The proportion of vegetables to noodles should be twice as many vegetables, or more, to noodles. You will have a nutrient-rich, low-calorie and low energy-dense meal, due to the high water content in the vegetables. Or, using our grapes and raisins example, a small bunch of red grapes will make you feel fuller, at a cost of far fewer calories, than will a handful of raisins. Compared to apple pie, an apple crisp or even a baked apple stuffed with 1 tablespoon of granola (which has a high energy density) and spices would be better, low energy-dense choices.

At the other extreme: cheese, chocolate, nuts, and chips are high energy-dense foods; their fat content is much higher than that of fresh fruits and vegetables. Some of these foods are nutrient-dense, and in some instances you should chose high energy-dense foods for their nutritional value. The trick is that you need to eat them in small portions. The avocado is a fine example, rich in healthy monounsaturated fats; the 45 calories in one ounce of succulent avocado flesh (roughly one-fourth of a medium-size avocado) will provide 6 percent of your daily values for vitamins E and B_6, magnesium, potassium, and fiber. It is, however, a high energy-dense food; hence, guacamole is energy-dense (and we never stop with just one tablespoon on two chips, do we? Try extending guacamole with chopped tomatoes, cilantro, and onions to dilute the density).

See the Food Data table on pages 170–189 for the energy density of foods. Keep in mind that what fills you up in the moment may not deter your hunger over a day as effectively as other types of foods. That is the challenge. Fats may take as long as five to seven hours to digest, proteins take up to four hours, and whole foods or complex carbohydrates take about two hours. Refined sugars pass through really quickly, in only thirty minutes. You will have to experiment a bit to see what suits your particular metabolism and lifestyle. For example, although fats log twice as many calories as carbohydrates, including them in your meals will slow the absorption of other foods, and will therefore help to stave off hunger. Likewise, adding a little protein to a largely carbohydrate meal will deter hunger longer. If you are a night owl who works deep into the wee hours, perhaps your dinnertime should be kicked back to a later hour and that meal contain primarily carbs, to provide you with the energy you need to keep going.

The Calorie Countdown

If you feel burdened by numbers and calculations, then proceed to the Weight Watcher section of this book, page 207. However, if you are a numbers person or a whiz on the computer, you just hit a home run: Following your natural inclination here will reward you with a satisfying transition into life on the Longevity Diet. Some members of the CR Society have designed their own interface to the USDA food database using Excel spreadsheets. Others make use of commercially available nutrition software programs.

What Should You Track? And How Often?

The following chapter will explain how to keep a journal of your meals and how to figure their calorie content. The calories, as well as nutritional content, of what you eat can be averaged over several days—the Longevity Diet is not about a struggle to get *precisely* 100 percent of *all* vitamins and minerals every single day. Beyond reducing your intake of calories, your priorities should be:

1. to eat enough protein for your body weight and level of CR (especially if you are a vegetarian)

2. to get adequate amounts of omega-3 fatty acids

3. to eliminate processed foods from your diet

Beyond that, eating enough fiber, low-GI carbohydrates, and foods rich in antioxidants should all be key elements of your Longevity Diet program. But these latter goals can make slow entrances, as you learn to eliminate unhealthy foods from your diet.

In the beginning, do your best to jettison all junk food, all empty calories. However, be compassionate with those moments of surrender to temptation, or the occasional meaningful splurge like a slice of birthday cake. The Longevity Diet is about saying yes to life; you can always make up for a cheese-and-wine sampler the next day with an especially high-nutrition, low-calorie meal. Indeed, in time you will find that a plate of colorful veggies is as much a yes to life as is a celebratory piece of cake with friends. Ultimately, CR can be seen as extending your food options, not restricting them. And it certainly extends your life!

If you are new to watching calories, it does help to read the labels on everything. Brand names, and even similar products produced by the same company, can vary widely in nutrient, fat, sodium, and sugar content. WestSoy, for example, markets regular soy milk, enriched soy milk, and low-fat soy milk. The enriched milk has almost twice the calories! If you include packaged foods in whatever CR program you use, compare the labels occasionally to see whether the manufacturer has changed any elements, particularly if a product has been repackaged as "improved."

Striking the Right Balance

- Fruits and veggies: Phytonutrient-rich foods *must* be included. Eat at least seven to nine servings of colorful fruits and vegetables per day, as described on pages 117–118.

- Omega-3 fatty acids: If you're not a vegetarian it is a good idea to eat at least two servings per week of a fatty fish, in particular, wild Atlantic or canned salmon, sardines, and herring. (As strange as it might sound, mash and eat the bones of canned salmon or sardines along with the fish, for extra calcium.) If you eat meat, choose 100 percent meat in low-fat cuts: lean red meats and pork, the light meat of poultry; avoid deli meats, frankfurters, "mystery meat" fast-food hamburgers, and bacon, all of which are rife with filler, chemicals, and fat. And eat some nuts (but not handfuls at one sitting!), especially walnuts and almonds, which are rich in healthy oils as well as important minerals.

- Healthy oils: When you cook with oils, use primarily mono-unsaturated fats, such as olive or canola oil. Eliminate trans-fatty acids from your diet; these are found in margarines, dressings, and deep-fried foods. (If you see "hydrogenated" in an ingredients list, the food has trans-fatty acids in it.)

- Calcium: Adequate calcium is especially important in the Longevity Diet; consider supplements, particularly if you avoid dairy products. Get into the habit of using skim or 2% milk rather than whole milk, and choose low-fat yogurts and cheeses. When selecting soy milks and yogurts, remember to read the ingredients label showing the vitamin and mineral content: some (even made by the same company) are more enriched than others.

- Choose whole grains over enriched grains: Choose whole wheat or multigrain artisan breads, brown rice rather than white rice, whole-grain pasta. Add legumes to your diet in the form of beans and peas, legume-based soups, peanut butter, hummus, soy products, and bean sprouts.

- Plant proteins: Don't neglect plant proteins if you're a vegetarian. Vegetarians should consider eating tempeh, seitan, calcium-fortified tofu, legumes, and low-fat soy products.

- Fiber: Adequate fiber is important: Choose whole foods over processed or refined foods, and do not overcook your grains and vegetables.

- Avoid sugars: Avoid foods high in refined sugar (watch out for corn syrup, pervasive in sweetened soft drinks and juices, even those sold in health food stores). Remember that, though natural, honey, maple syrup, brown rice syrup, and other sweeteners are essentially just sugar.

LOUISE AND RODNEY

When asked if there is a skillful way to practice CR, Louise said that you should be mindful, respect your body, and be aware of what kind of nutrition you personally need. She and her partner, Peter Voss, have been practicing the lifestyle for many years. When I visited them for this interview, Peter mentioned that the whole point is to change habits from destructive unconscious health choices to good ones. He proceeded to serve himself a breakfast with strawberries, papaya, mango, raspberries, and grapes!

Louise says: How did I start? I decided to watch what I was eating, and learn how many calories were in my food. I used to work at the Hilton Corporate office, and they baked fresh scones every morning. So I would begin my morning with a cup of coffee and a scone, and I thought that it was a good breakfast because the scone has blueberries! I thought that a scone only had 150 calories. One day I weighed one, and realized that that single scone was about 500 calories. Once I found out, I let the scones go. Occasionally I will still have one, but not every day! So I was becoming aware of the calories.

Peter and I started keeping a food diary of everything we ate, and we looked up the calorie content of everything. In the beginning Peter was measuring our food, so I became aware of how much an ounce was, and what a portion size was. That also helped me realize how many calories I was really eating. It would drive me crazy, though, to weigh food,

I cannot do that now! Some people need to do it, but I now know what 4 ounces of salmon looks like, or 4 ounces of filet mignon! I don't want it to interfere with my life!

Peter and I have diverged on our strategies, as Peter became an enthusiast of eating small meals, and I prefer two ample meals a day. When he consumes small meals, he doesn't get hungry, nor does he think about food. There are so many ways to practice, but we eat differently.

Some people can graze, some people fast one day a week, some eat one large meal a day. You have to find out what works for you, what the demands of your life are, and what you have the time for. Grazing takes more time. Personally, I need to feel somewhat full after eating to be satisfied.

Rodney says:

CR doesn't seem to be particularly difficult so far. Perhaps snacking after 7:00 p.m. is something I would like to get better under control. An automatic timed lock on the refrigerator door that unlocks at 6:00 a.m. and locks at 7:00 p.m. might help? Sounds a bit draconian, but might be worth trying!

I started CR quite gradually, by exerting marginally more control over my caloric intake than I was used to. The result has been a weight loss of about half a pound a week. The quality of my diet has always been good, so I tried to cut back on calories by eating fewer starches. I learned what I could to further improve the quality of my meals: I started eating lots of soups, especially homemade, containing all the foods believed to be the healthiest, whether or not the conventional wisdom believes they belong in soup! Multiple vegetable; tomato; miso; commercial chicken noodle with green vegetables added; bean and pea. I avoid fats in general, trans fats and cancer-implicated oils in particular. And I eat at least some fish pretty much every day, 90 percent of it canned—salmon, mackerel, sardines, tuna, or herring.

7
Your Daily Food Diary

Let's face it, your relationship to food is one of the most basic relationships that you have. In the very first phase of your life, the milk in your mother's breast was the simple answer to your body's most pressing nutritional needs. Not long thereafter, life became much more complicated. With life's complications came food on the run, food from machines, instant or processed food, school cafeteria and restaurant food, and party food.

Food can calm you when you are under duress; it can also relate powerful feelings to others—cooking something sensual for a romantic partner, generously providing a magnificent spread for family or friends. To many people, food represents bonding with the people closest to you, a literal reassertion of how well you understand each other's tastes. From the moment you left your mother's milk behind, food has been about far more than simply satisfying your hunger.

In this chapter you will learn to separate what you eat from all the extra meanings and circumstances that surround it, by keeping a diary that makes you conscious of what you are ingesting, and when. Unlike life, there is nothing complicated about it: this diary is intentionally straightforward, to enable you to use it unhesitatingly and, though consciously, un*self*-consciously. When you know that you will be reviewing later what you write down today, this awareness shall eventually inspire you to make better food choices—or, at least more thoughtful ones. Be patient with yourself—you will be the only person reading this diary, and if you slip every so often with a large meal or sugary snack, consider such slips useful information about behaviors that could still use some attention.

While you record what you eat and drink, think about (perhaps even jot down) the influences that may have affected your dining decisions: emotional triggers, what people were eating in your presence, and other situations that tend to push you into reactive or mechanical patterns. For example, consider restaurant dining: do you habitually fill up on bread as you wait for the meal you ordered to be prepared for you, even if it means taking home a "doggy bag" of a main dish you then cannot finish? Do you feel obligated to have an appetizer if not ordering one would make you the only person at the table without one? As you notice such tendencies, your diary will help prepare you to change your dietary behaviors to saying no or making substitutions, ultimately consuming only those foods that will do your body the most good.

Do not think about calories at this point. If you get obsessed about numerical details in the beginning, you may overlook the sensory pleasures of eating wholesome foods, which is what this diet is all about. A week after you begin the diary, you will consider the nutritional content of what you normally consume, and then finally its caloric content. But for now, for one week you will simply write down your meals and snacks . . . your baseline diet.

Start by writing down everything you eat and drink. Yes, *everything,* even if it's just a cracker with your soup or a glass of milk before bedtime. There is no rigid format as to how to keep your diary; if you are a grazer rather than a three-meals-per-day person, ignore the meal/snack headings in the chart that follows and just write down what you eat at what hour. The important thing is to remember to write everything down. The times of day do become an important factor later along, as they will help you figure out which mealtimes or snack times are more habitual than nutrient-necessary for you, as well as which kinds of nutrients your body seems to crave at certain hours.

HELGA

Helga's transition into what she calls her "plant-based diet" was itself almost organic. She explained to us that she needed to actually see the meals and the food before she was convinced that it was something worth trying. Fortunately, she was close friends with Lisa's father, and experienced firsthand his savory concoctions, such as Eternal Youth Chili (recipe included).

Helga says: I basically have two meals a day. I have my shake in the morning of several kinds of fruit, whey protein, Udo's Choice Oil Blend, and a little milk or yogurt. I usually do not eat lunch. Then in the evening I have steamed veggies every other day and eat the leftovers the next day. I love potatoes, my comfort food, this stems from my childhood, and I add a little olive oil. I might make a salad with avocado and cherry tomatoes, sometimes rice. I love whole-grain bread, and I eat salmon twice a week, and turkey. I prefer low-level animal protein, as I got into a lot of trouble with low B12. I did not know I was anemic and had a hard time getting around. I have good control over things now and I have plenty of energy.

I have always liked vegetables and fish. I never felt that I was walking around starving. My favorite meal is brown rice and black beans with lots of steamed vegetables doused with olive oil—that is like mother's milk! I am still learning about nutrition all the time.

I don't think it would work for me if I was starving myself. I would have to be comfortable, and I was, so CR was not difficult for me.

A typical day's jottings before engaging in the Longevity Lifestyle might look like this:

DAILY FOOD DIARY
Begin by keeping simple lists of everything you eat during the days

DAY OF THE WEEK: _____ **TIME**

BREAKFAST

_____

_____

_____

_____

_____

MORNING SNACK

_____

LUNCH

_____

_____

_____

_____

AFTERNOON SNACK

_____

DINNER

_____

_____

_____

_____

EVENING SNACK

_____

_____

DAILY FOOD DIARY

DAY OF THE WEEK:	TIME
BREAKFAST	*7:30*
2 scrambled eggs with 2 slices bacon	
1 cup orange juice	
English muffin with 2 tablespoons butter	
black coffee	
MORNING SNACK	*11:00*
Starbucks maple scone	
Starbucks coffee Frappuccino	
LUNCH	*1:00*
hamburger (single patty on bun) with slice of tomato, ketchup, and mayo	
3 oz. French fries	
10 oz. Coca-Cola	
AFTERNOON SNACK	*4:00*
1 oz. peanuts	
banana	
black coffee	
DINNER	*8:00*
cocktail; 12 oz. beer	
6 crackers with cheese	
1 cup lentil soup	
dinner roll with butter	
1 glass (8 oz.) white wine	
3 oz. broiled salmon with tartar sauce	
½ cup carrots	
¾ cup mashed potatoes	
EVENING SNACK	*10:30*
apple pie with 1 scoop ice cream	
1 cup milk	

Tracking Your Nutrients

Once you have recorded a week's worth of meals, transfer your diary notations into the Nutrition Tracker that follows, using our breakdown below to note which nutritional factors, such as protein or calcium, compose each of the foods and beverages you have recorded. Some individual foods or a dish involving several ingredients may bridge more than one category, in which case you will need to check off all appropriate categories for that food. For instance, salmon contains both protein and omega-3; if you have lentil soup and crackers, you would check off both protein and whole grains (lentils), and enriched grains (crackers). If you have a nutrition software program (see Resources), use it to help you monitor the nutritional value of your selected foods and beverages.

How to List Foods and Beverages in the Nutrient Tracker

1. **Vegetables and Fruits:** vegetables and fruits, 100 percent vegetable and fruit juices, and vegetable products, such as tomato sauce.
2. **Whole Grains:** whole grains and whole-grain products, legumes.
3. **Protein:** eggs, poultry, fish, meat, nuts, soy products, legumes, cheese.
4. **Omega-3:** salmon, sardines, and coldwater fish; olive or canola oil; flaxseeds; walnuts; avocados.
5. **Fats:** hydrogenated polyunsaturated fats (most margarines and dressings); monounsaturated fats from meat, poultry, or dairy sources (such as butter); rich sauces.
6. **Calcium:** dairy products, soy and tofu, dark green leafy vegetables, fish eaten with their soft bones (such as canned salmon or sardines).

7. **Enriched Foods and Sweets:** enriched grains such as white rice, and enriched-grain products: most cereals, crackers, pasta, breads, processed and fast foods—any food high in corn syrup, which is pervasive in commercial brands—most dairy desserts and baked desserts, granulated sugar and honey, jams and jellies, candy, soft drinks, and non–100 percent juice drinks such as cranberry juice cocktail and spritzers.

8. **Miscellaneous:** condiments such as ketchup, prepared mustard, salsa, jam; beverages such as tea, coffee, seltzer water, and water.

NUTRITION TRACKER

List each food from your daily food journal and place it in the proper column(s).

TODAY'S DATE:

FOODS YOU ATE TODAY	VEGETABLES & FRUIT	WHOLE GRAINS & WHOLE GRAIN PRODUCTS	PROTEIN	OMEGA-3 FOODS & FATS

FATS	CALCIUM FOODS	ENRICHED OR FAST FOODS & SWEETS	MISC.	CALORIES

Here's how our meal example would add up:

NUTRITION TRACKER

List each food from your daily food journal and place it in the proper column(s).

TODAY'S DATE:

FOODS YOU ATE TODAY	VEGETABLES & FRUIT	WHOLE GRAINS & WHOLE GRAIN PRODUCTS	PROTEIN	OMEGA-3 FOODS & FATS
Breakfast, 7:30	8 oz. orange juice	English muffin	2 scrambled eggs 2 slices bacon	
Morning Snack, 11:00		Starbucks maple scone		
Lunch, 1:00	slice tomato		hamburger patty	
Afternoon Snack, 4:00	banana		1 oz. peanuts	
Cocktail, 7:15			cheese	
Dinner, 8:00	¾ cup mashed potatoes ½ cup carrots lentil soup		1 cup lentil soup 3 oz. salmon	
Evening Snack	apple pie			

But What About Calories?

The final step in structuring your food diary—once you have become familiar with the nutrients of the foods you eat, and have perhaps already begun selecting foods that can be listed in the healthier categories—is to begin calculating how many calories you are consuming per portion size. Packaged foods usually in-

FATS	CALCIUM FOODS	ENRICHED OR FAST FOODS & SWEETS	MISC.	CALORIES
2 tsp. butter			coffee	
			Starbucks coffee Frappuccino	
mayonnaise		white bread bun 3 oz. French fries ketchup (sugar) 10 oz. Coca-Cola		
			coffee	
		12 oz. beer crackers		
2 tsp. butter tartar sauce ¼ cup milk (in potatoes)	2 tsp. butter	dinner roll with butter	8 oz. white wine	
	1 scoop ice cream	apple pie 1 scoop ice cream		

clude the calorie count per serving on the area of the package that contains ingredient information. Do take portion size seriously: a cup of a particular fresh vegetable, such as steamed kale, may be considerably more than you are accustomed to eating, and if you eat less, the calories you list for it need to be lowered accordingly; on the other hand, when you fill your bowl with breakfast cereal, you may be eating far more than the serving size suggested on the side box panel that contains its calorie information. This goes for every food down the list: If you've never actually measured your servings, it might be helpful for you to weigh your food on a food scale or pour into a measuring cup the amounts that the calorie chart or package label specifies as a serving. Don't worry, you won't be measuring food your whole life! After a while you will be able to eyeball the correct amount. You'll get used to

NUTRITION TRACKER

List each food from your daily food journal and place it in the proper column(s).

TODAY'S DATE:

FOODS YOU ATE TODAY	VEGETABLES & FRUIT	WHOLE GRAINS & WHOLE GRAIN PRODUCTS	PROTEIN	OMEGA-3 FOODS & FATS
Breakfast, 7:30	8 oz. orange juice	English muffin	2 scrambled eggs 2 slices bacon	
Morning Snack, 11:00		Starbucks maple scone		
Lunch, 1:00	slice tomato		hamburger patty	
Afternoon Snack, 4:00	banana		1 oz. peanuts	
Cocktail, 7:15			cheese	
Dinner, 8:00	¾ cup mashed potatoes ¼ cup carrots lentil soup		1 cup lentil soup 3 oz. salmon	
Evening Snack	apple pie			

the idea that a healthy serving of fish, poultry, or meat should not exceed the size of the palm of your hand.

Once you become familiar with what constitutes a portion and standardize how much you typically consume, filling the calories into your Nutrient Tracker will become a simple matter of looking up what calories you listed for that food when you last ate it.

When you are ready to include the calorie count of your foods, fill in the last column on the Nutrient Tracker on pages 142–143. Our sample meal would add up as follows:

FATS	CALCIUM FOODS	ENRICHED OR FAST FOODS & SWEETS	MISC.	CALORIES
2 tsp. butter			coffee	630
			Starbucks coffee Frappuccino	550
mayonnaise		white bread bun 3 oz. French fries ketchup (sugar) 10 oz. Coca-Cola		1,000
			coffee	240
		12 oz. beer crackers		460
2 tsp. butter tartar sauce ¼ cup milk (in potatoes)	2 tsp. butter	dinner roll with butter	8 oz. white wine	850
	1 scoop ice cream	apple pie 1 scoop ice cream		500
			TOTAL	4,233

What a CR Daily Food Diary Might Look Like

As you will see from the following example, Lisa eats her main meal at night. Her intake reflects her profile. She is a petite—under five feet tall and weighing eighty pounds—vegetarian. From the list below, she made the assessment that her diet was a little

LISA'S NUTRITION TRACKER

List each food from your daily food journal and place it in the proper column(s).

TODAY'S DATE:

FOODS YOU ATE TODAY	VEGETABLES & FRUIT	WHOLE GRAINS & WHOLE GRAIN PRODUCTS	PROTEIN	OMEGA-3 FOODS & FATS
breakfast			4 walnuts, 6 almonds, 10 peanuts	walnuts
morning snack	1" avocado slice	½ slice whole wheat toast	2 tbsp. hummus spread (chickpeas)	1" avocado slice
midafternoon snack	16 oz. apple/ beet/carrot juice			
dinner	Steamed: broccoli, red pepper, kale, tomato, squash, sweet potato, onions, cauliflower ½ cup tomato sauce		2 oz. baked tofu	1 tsp. olive oil 1 tsp. flax oil
evening snack			10 toasted almonds	

low in protein, and was high in heart-healthy fats. You will see she recorded everything she ate, even if it was only a light snack.

Lisa's food list includes these serving totals by category: approximately 10 servings of veggies and fruits; protein, 4 servings; omega-3, 3 servings; fats, 3 servings; calcium, 4 servings. She takes calcium and B_{12} supplements.

FATS	CALCIUM FOODS	ENRICHED OR FAST FOODS & SWEETS	MISC.	CALORIES
			black tea	
	2 oz. baked tofu		black pepper marjoram	

As You Begin the Longevity Diet

Now that you understand how to keep a Daily Food Diary, use it (page 139), along with the Nutrient Tracker on pages 142–143, to record the foods and beverages that you consume. Refer to chapter 6 for ways to improve the nutritional content of your intake while reducing such unhealthy elements as processed carbs, and chart your progress.

Don't despair if the record-keeping feels complicated at first; once you become accustomed to viewing your foods with an eye toward their categories, keeping the lists will become much easier. Indeed, as you become comfortable with what constitutes healthy foods, you will enjoy finding ever more creative ways to keep clear of the "unhealthy" columns, as well as to nip and tuck your calorie intake. Think of making substitutions as playing a game in which the lowest scores advance you toward the winner's box: each week, try to beat last week's low calorie count, or to keep from eating anything that would require you to place a check in an "unhealthy" column. For instance, if you find yourself at a food court, opting for sushi or all-veggie fajitas would be the way to go, rather than heading for the burger counter—bing! you won that round! Remember to eat something supernutritious to make up for any slips into the high yet nutritionally empty calorie columns. Whatever you do, keep in mind that your goal is not to write down less and less *food*, but to eat a satisfying quantity and range of nutritious, low-calorie foods fitting into as many *healthy* categories as possible.

Helga told us, "Plugging your calories into a program was a difficult idea; most people do not want a laptop in their kitchen. But when you internalize it, you don't need any of those gadgets. And once you get going, I don't think you need to count calories. It won't be a thing that impinges on your lifestyle."

Here are examples of four different approaches to following the Longevity Diet. The first traces a meal plan for a middle-aged woman who is moderately active and transitioning to healthier eating. You will see a turkey sandwich, halibut, hot chocolate, and brandy. The second example is Brian's meal calendar. Brian is in his forties, moderately active, and has been following the Longevity Diet for over fifteen years. He eats two solid meals a day, featuring fruits, vegetables, grains, and protein (legumes or fish). The Grazer eats many small meals throughout the day to satisfy his or her needs. This plan is for a middle-aged woman who is moderately active. And finally, take a look at a nutritious vegetarian. This plan is for a middle-aged woman who is moderately active. Men would add approximately five hundred calories to these figures, depending on activity level and desired calorie restriction. There is no right way or best way; there is the way that will work for you!

These daily meal plans reach close to 100 percent for most of the recommended dietary allowance (RDA) for vitamins and minerals. The RDA is the average daily dietary intake level that is sufficient to meet the nutrient requirements of nearly all healthy individuals. Remember, these figures are baseline values meant to prevent deficiencies. After reviewing our material and educating yourself a little on the nutritional needs of your body, you may decide to increase some baseline values.

We have included total values for protein, fiber, and fat, along with the percent of RDA values for a few key vitamins and minerals.

HEALTHY CHOICES THREE-MEAL-A-DAY PLAN—DAY ONE

(Figures based on basic Recommended Dietary Allowances for a middle-aged woman who is moderately active; men add 500 calories)

AMOUNT	FOOD ITEM	CALORIES
BREAKFAST		
12 oz	Coffee	7
1 cup	Low-fat milk (in coffee or cereal)	119
1 pack	Oatmeal, multigrain	60
1 tbs	Walnuts	50
SNACK		
1 cup	Nonfat cottage cheese	160
⅓ cup	Mandarin oranges, canned, juice packed	45
LUNCH		
2 slices	Whole wheat bread	120
2 oz	Turkey breast, white meat, roasted	100
½	Tomato, sliced	6
1 tbs	Dijon mustard	3
leaf	Romaine lettuce	3
16 oz	Tea, green or black	10
SNACK		
8	Carrots, mini snack pack	24
½ cup	Hummus	200
1 cup	Spicy tomato juice	41
DINNER		
5 oz	Halibut	150
1 cup	Mixed vegetables	100
½ tbs	Olive oil (over vegetables)	60
1 small	Green salad, lettuce, cucumbers, tomato	44
1 tbs	Commercial salad dressing	70
½ cup	Red wine	74
SNACK (hot chocolate with brandy)		
1 cup	Lowfat milk	100
1 tbs	Cocoa, unsweetened	40
1 oz	Brandy or other liqueur	100
TOTAL		*1,503*

Calories per day: 1,503

Percent of calories from:
Protein: 30
Carbohydrate: 47
Fat: 23
Total protein: 111 gm
Total fiber: 18 gm
Total cholesterol: 124 mg

Total fat: 38 g
%Saturated: 48
%Monounsaturated: 54
%Polyunsaturated: 158

Nutritional Profile
Percent of RDA per serving based on an average
2,000 calorie a day:
Vitamin A: 419
Vitamin C: 251
Vitamin E: 102
Vitamin B_{12}: 254
Iron: 68
Calcium: 96
Selenium: 213
Magnesium: 153
Zinc: 71
Potassium: 184
Niacin: 132
Folic Acid: 182

Adequate protein (55–65 gm);
adequate fiber (40–60 gm)

HEALTHY CHOICES THREE-MEAL-A-DAY PLAN—DAY TWO

(Figures based on basic Recommended Dietary Allowances for a woman who is moderately active; men add 500 calories)

AMOUNT	FOOD ITEM	CALORIES
BREAKFAST		
12 oz	Coffee or tea	5
1 cup	Low-fat milk (in coffee or cereal)	120
1 pack	1 egg, poached or hard boiled	75
1 tbs	1 slice multi-grain toast	70
1 pat, 5 gm	butter	35
SNACK		
1	Medium apple	80
1 oz	Almonds	165
LUNCH		
1	Pita pocket, whole wheat	75
2 oz	Tuna salad, commercially prepared	100
½	Tomato, sliced	6
leaf	Romaine lettuce	3
1	Onion slice	3
16 oz	Tea, green or black, or soda water with 2 oz orange juice, natural orange soda (35 calories total)	5
SNACK		
3 cups	Popcorn, air-popped	90
1 cup	Spicy tomato juice	40
DINNER		
5 oz	Enchilada:	
1	Corn tortilla	60
½ cup	Mixed frozen vegetables, red bell peppers	50
½ cup	Refried black beans	110
1 oz	Low-fat cheddar cheese	50
½ cup	Enchilada sauce, commercial brand	60
1	Tomato, sliced, alongside enchilada	20
½ cup	Brown rice, cooked and mixed with a little salsa	110
1 cup	Green salad, lettuce	8
1 tbs	Carrot, sliced or grated in salad	10
12 oz	Beer	135
SNACK		
1 oz	Dark chocolate	150
TOTAL		*1,635*

Calories per day: 1,635

Percent of calories from:
Protein: 16
Carbohydrate: 55
Fat: 29
Total protein: 62 gm
Total fiber: 33 gm
Total cholesterol: 250 mg

Total fat: 52 g
%Saturated: 78
%Monounsaturated: 74
%Polyunsaturated: 167

Nutritional Profile
Percent of RDA per serving based on an average
2,000 calorie a day:
Vitamin A: 289
Vitamin C: 255
Vitamin E: 124
Vitamin B_{12}: 83
Iron: 93
Calcium: 45
Selenium: 180
Magnesium: 153
Zinc: 75
Potassium: 155
Niacin: 119
Folic acid: 204

Adequate protein (55–65 gm);
adequate fiber (40–60 gm)

LONGEVITY LIFESTYLE VETERAN TWO-MEAL-A-DAY PLAN—DAY ONE

(Figures based on basic Recommended Dietary Allowances for a middle-aged man who has been practicing CR for over 10 years)

AMOUNT	FOOD ITEM	CALORIES
BREAKFAST		
1 cup	Coffee or tea	5
1 cup	Bowl of cereal: oatmeal	260
.5 oz	Raisins	40
1	Banana	90
¼ cup	Soymilk	30
½ cup	Frozen blueberries	20
½ cup	Nonfat yogurt	45
3	Walnuts, whole, chopped up	50
SNACK		
1	Apple	80
1 tbs	Peanut butter, smeared on apple slices	95
DINNER		
3 oz	Salmon	175
½ cup	Wild rice	80
¼ cup	Red pepper puree sauce on rice	50
1 cup	Kale	40
1 stalk	Carrot	25
1 stalk	Broccoli	50
1 cup	Seasonal fruit, melon, berries	60
2 tsp	Olive oil	70
1 oz	Very dark chocolate	150
6 oz	Red wine	125
TOTAL		*1,540*

Calories per day: 1,540

Percent of calories from:
Protein:
Carbohydrate: 64
Fat: 23
Total protein: 59 gm
Total fiber: 27 gm
Total cholesterol: 55 mg

Total fat: 52 g
%Saturated: 61
%Monounsaturated: 79
%Polyunsaturated: 197

Nutritional Profile
percent of RDA per serving based on an average
2,000 calorie a day:
Vitamin A: 647
Vitamin C: 536
Vitamin E: 166
Vitamin B_{12}: 157
Iron: 123
Calcium: 69
Selenium: 128
Magnesium: 150
Zinc: 62
Potassium: 183
Niacin: 156
Folic acid: 299

Adequate protein (55–65 gm);
adequate fiber (40–60 gm)

LONGEVITY LIFESTYLE VETERAN TWO-MEAL-A-DAY PLAN—DAY TWO

(Figures based on basic Recommended Dietary Allowances for a middle-aged man who has been practicing CR for over 10 years)

AMOUNT	FOOD ITEM	CALORIES
BREAKFAST		
1	Large apple	125
1 ½ cup	Large bowl of cereal: Kamut	210
¼ cup	Oats	180
.5 oz	Raisins	40
¼ cup	Soymilk	30
½ cup	Frozen blueberries	20
¼ cup	Nonfat yogurt	30
25	Almonds	150
SNACK		
¾ cup	Strawberries (about 10)	60
½ oz	Cashews	80
DINNER (large bowl of stew)		
½ cup	Cooked pinto beans (or other legume)	120
½ cup	Brown rice (or other grain)	105
1 small	Sweet potato (beets)	55
1 stalk	Broccoli, large (or other green vege)	80
1 cup	Watermelon (in season, or other fruit)	45
1	Nectarine	55
1 oz	Very dark chocolate	150
6 oz	Red wine	125
TOTAL		**1,660**

Calories per day: 1,660

Percent of calories from:
Protein: 13
Carbohydrate: 65
Fat: 22
Total protein: 53 gm
Total fiber: 46 gm
Total cholesterol: 1 mg

Total fat: 39 g
%Saturated: 47
%Monounsaturated: 63
%Polyunsaturated: 123

Nutritional Profile:
percent of RDA per serving based on an average
2,000 calorie a day:
Vitamin A: 433
Vitamin C: 386
Vitamin E: 165
Vitamin B_{12}: 18
Iron: 108
Calcium: 47
Selenium: 141
Magnesium: 208
Zinc: 87
Potassium: 171
Niacin: 73
Folic acid: 225

LONGEVITY VETERAN GRAZER MEAL PLAN
(MANY SMALL MEALS A DAY) — DAY ONE
(Figures based on basic Recommended Dietary Allowances for a middle-aged woman who is moderately active; men add 500 calories)

AMOUNT	FOOD ITEM	CALORIES
EARLY AM MEAL		
12 oz	Tea with 1 oz skim milk	10
7	Large strawberries	40
10	Raspberries	10
REPEAT EARLY AM MEAL		60
1ST MORNING SNACK		
1	Large carrot	25
5	Almonds	50
2ND SNACK		
12 oz	Tea with 1 oz skim milk	10
7	Strawberries	40
Small bunch	Grapes	10
2ND SNACK		
Approx 2 oz each	Broccoli, cauliflower, asparagus, carrot, zucchini, spinach, mushrooms, sweet potato, tomato, raw purple cabbage, cucumber (rainbow)	350
3 tbs	Follow-your-heart salad dressing	170
SNACK		
¼	Small avocado	75
1 oz	Cheddar cheese	50
DINNER		
¼ oz	Flaxseed	30
1ST AFTERNOON SNACK		
12 oz	Tea	10
½	Small papaya	30
½	Each kiwi, persimmon	100
2ND SNACK		
2	Low-fat cracker	50
2 tsp	Peanut butter	90
⅓	Banana	50

EARLY EVENING SNACK		
12 oz	Tea with skim milk	10
¼ cup	Blueberries	20
5	Strawberries	25
¼	Apple	50
MID EVENING SNACK		
7	Strawberries	40
2 oz	Dark chocolate	200
TOTAL		1,605

Calories per day: 1,605

Percent of calories from:
Protein:
Carbohydrate:
Fat:
Total protein 50 gm
Total fiber: 66 gm
Total cholesterol: 25 mg

Total fat: 66 g
%Saturated: 100
%Monounsaturated: 82
%Polyunsaturated: 253

Nutritional Profile:
percent of RDA per serving based on an average
2,000 calorie a day:
Vitamin A: 1,490
Vitamin C: 1,035
Vitamin E: 220
Vitamin B_{12}: 30
Iron: 124
Calcium: 79
Selenium: 63
Magnesium: 240
Zinc: 76
Potassium: 315
Niacin: 95
Folic acid: 463

Adequate protein (55–65 gm);
adequate fiber (40–60 gm)

LONGEVITY VETERAN GRAZER MEAL PLAN
(MANY SMALL MEALS A DAY) — DAY TWO
(Figures based on basic Recommended Dietary Allowances for a middle-aged woman who is moderately active; men add 500 calories)

AMOUNT	FOOD ITEM	CALORIES
AM MEAL		
12 oz	Tea	4
1	Apple	75
1 cup	Blueberries, frozen, thawed	80
MID MORNING		
1 cup	Cooked quinoa	158
12	Almonds, chopped	84
LATE MORNING		
12 oz	Tea	4
1 cup	Nonfat cottage cheese	160
1	Crispbread cracker, or 3 Ak-Mak, Ryvita	100
1 cup	Applesauce	100
PM MEAL		
2 slices	Steamed vegetables or salad	120
1 stalk	Broccoli	65
2	Tomatoes	25
4	Mushrooms	15
1 medium	Zucchini squash	30
1 cup	Cauliflower	30
½ medium	Sweet potato	55
1 small	Sweet red pepper	35
2 tbs	Fat-free salad dressing	26
2 oz	Salmon	100
1 tsp	Ground flaxseed	20
EARLY EVENING		
1	Banana	90
2 tbs	Peanut butter	190
8 oz	Green tea	
LATE EVENING		
3 cups	Air-popped popcorn	90
TOTAL		*1,656*

Calories per day: 1,656

Percent of calories from:
Protein:
Carbohydrate:
Fat:
Total protein 88 gm
Total fiber: 55 gm
Total cholesterol: 49 mg

Total fat: 38 g
%Saturated: 34
%Monounsaturated: 54
%Polyunsaturated: 173

Nutritional Profile:
percent of RDA per serving based on an average
2,000 calorie a day:
Vitamin A: 1,088
Vitamin C: 1,010
Vitamin E: 306
Vitamin B_{12}: 361
Iron: 195
Calcium: 64
Selenium: 177
Magnesium: 212
Zinc: 128
Potassium: 271
Niacin: 187
Folic acid: 382

VEGETARIAN THREE-MEAL-
A-DAY PLAN) — DAY ONE

(Figures based on basic Recommended Dietary Allowances for a middle-aged woman who is moderately active; men add 500 calories)

AMOUNT	FOOD ITEM	CALORIES
BREAKFAST		
12 oz	Tea or coffee	7
¼ cup	Soy milk (in coffee or cereal)	20
¼ cup	Wheat germ	100
¼ each	Apple, banana, orange, other fruit, 1 ½ cup total	151
1/2 cup	Non fat yogurt (or soy)	68
SNACK		
1 oz	Almonds	160
1 cup	Tea	
LUNCH		
1	Whole wheat pita pocket	74
2	Falafel patties	110
½	Tomato, sliced	6
2 tbs	Hummus	46
leaf	Romaine lettuce or sprouts	3
16 oz	Tea, green or black	10
SNACK		
8	Carrots, mini snack pack	24
1 oz	Pretzels, whole wheat	100
1 cup	Soy, almond, or rice milk, flavored	120
DINNER		
1 ½ cup	Scrambled tofu	150
½ cup	Mixed vegetables	50
1 tbs	Olive oil (over vegetables and to cook tofu)	120
½ cup	Brown rice, cooked	110
¼ cup	Wild rice, cooked	40
½ cup	Red wine or concord grape juice	74
SNACK		
1 cup	Non-fat yogurt	100
1 tbs	Oatmeal cookie or fruit	92
TOTAL		**1,600**

Calories per day: 1,600

Percent of calories from:
Protein: 18
Carbohydrate: 51
Fat: 31
Total protein 74 gm
Total fiber: 34 gm
Total cholesterol: 6 mg

Total fat: 55 g
%Saturated: 39
%Monounsaturated: 96
%Polyunsaturated: 253

Nutritional Profile:
percent of RDA per serving based on an average
2,000 calorie a day:
Vitamin A: 137
Vitamin C: 385
Vitamin E: 191
Vitamin B_{12}: 113
Iron: 89
Calcium: 84
Selenium: 144
Magnesium: 333
Zinc: 114
Potassium: 195
Niacin: 86
Folic acid: 222

Adequate protein (55–65 gm);
adequate fiber (40–60 gm)

VEGETARIAN THREE-MEAL-
A-DAY PLAN) — DAY TWO

(Figures based on basic Recommended Dietary Allowances for a middle-aged woman who is moderately active; men add 500 calories)

AMOUNT	FOOD ITEM	CALORIES
BREAKFAST		
1 cup	Tea or coffee	5
	Smoothie:	
1 cup	Soy milk (or skim milk)	100
½ cup	Nonfat yogurt (or soy)	65
1 small	Banana	90
1 cup	Strawberries	45
SNACK		
About 10	Almonds	80
1 cup	Tea	
LUNCH (Big salad)		
½ cup each	Broccoli, cauliflower, carrot (1 cup), zucchini, spinach, mushrooms, celery, red pepper, tomato, raw purple cabbage, cucumber (rainbow)	200
1 tbs	Olive oil	115
1 tsp	Balsamic vinegar	15
2 tsp	Sunflower seeds	90
2 tbs	Hummus	46
¼	Avocado	75
1 slice	Whole wheat toast	70
16 oz	Tea, green or black	5
SNACK		
1 oz	Pretzels, whole wheat	100
1 cup	Soy, almond, or rice milk, flavored (chai tea)	120
DINNER		
½ cup	Indian lentils (dahl) with spices	115
½ cup each	Brown rice, prepared Indian style, Biryani, with peas and carrots and spices	140
1 cup	Mustard greens or spinach pureed with	30
¼ cup	Non-fat yogurt (or soy)	35
½ cup	Red wine or concord grape juice	75
TOTAL		*1,616*

Calories per day: 1,616

Percent of calories from:
Protein: 19
Carbohydrate: 50
Fat: 30
Total protein 74 gm
Total fiber: 56 gm
Total cholesterol: 5 mg

Total fat: 56 g
%Saturated: 39
%Monounsaturated: 86
%Polyunsaturated: 277

Nutritional Profile:
percent of RDA per serving based on an average
2,000 calorie a day:
Vitamin A: 1,448
Vitamin C: 889
Vitamin E: 246
Vitamin B$_{12}$: 65
Iron: 161
Calcium: 100
Selenium: 113
Magnesium: 248
Zinc: 96
Potassium: 347
Niacin: 125
Folic acid: 650

Adequate protein (55–65 gm);
adequate fiber (40–60 gm)

Following is a table of foods and beverages, listing their calories per serving size, and also the degree to which they are nutritious (energy density). Again, don't be intimidated by this degree of information. In time, you will learn which foods have similar numbers, and will be able to make healthy everyday dining selections without always needing to consult the charts. For more information, you might also wish to visit these Web sites:

http://is.gd/4KwKC is the shortcut for www.photosmash.net/ Usda_data/foods_db.html. This is a companion piece to this book, attached to Dr. Walford's Web site. It is a search engine that delivers almost everything you need to know about more than five thousand foods—vitamins, minerals, and the percentage of calories from fat, protein, and carbohydrates are all listed in an accessible format.

In addition, the search engine is a highly informative extension of the basic search engine on Walford.com that allows you to compare and identify foods that are highest or lowest in twenty-eight nutrient categories. However, please note that it does not feature many name-brand foods.[1]

http://spaz.ca/cronometer/ is a free, open source and cross-platform dieting program. Along with the basics of tracking your nutritional profile over one or several days, preparing recipes, sharing data and recipes, Cronometer also allows you to track and chart your biometrics.[2]

www.nutritiondata.com/tools/nutrient-search allows you to search the USDA food database to find foods that are highest or lowest in particular nutrients. For instance, you could look for foods that are rich in calcium and low in calories. [3]

www.nal.usda.gov/fnic/foodcomp/search/index.html is the most comprehensive site, albeit a bit unwieldy. It even includes a complete lipid breakdown, i.e., what kinds of fats are in each food.[4]

FOOD DATA TABLE

FOOD	SERVING SIZE	CALORIES	GRAMS	ENERGY DENSITY (cal/gr) Choose low values
VEGETABLES				
Artichokes	Base ends & leaves	26	100	0.3
Asparagus	4 large spears	24	100	0.2
Beet Greens	1 cup, cooked	40	150	0.3
Beets	1 cup, diced	60	140	0.4
Broccoli	1 medium stalk	50	180	0.3
Brussels Sprouts	2 large	59	140	0.4
Cabbage	1 cup, finely shredded	23	90	0.3
Cabbage, Chinese (napa)	1 cup, 1-inch pieces	9	75	0.1
Cabbage, Red	1 cup, shredded	27	100	0.3
Carrots	1 carrot (7½″ × 1⅛″)	35	80	0.4
Cauliflower	1 cup florets	25	100	0.3
Celeriac	¼ of one large	42	100	0.4
Celery	1 cup, chopped	19	120	0.2
Chard	¼ lb.	21	115	0.2
Corn	kernels of 1 cob (5″ × 1¾″)	110	140	0.8
Corn	½ cup frozen prepared	65	82	0.8
Cucumber	1 small (6″ × 1½″)	21	180	0.1
Eggplant	1 cup, diced	56	200	0.3
Garlic	1 clove (1½″ × ½″ × ⅓″)	5	3	1.7
Kale	¼ lb.	32	115	0.3
Leeks	3 to 4 (5″)	31	100	0.3
Lettuce, Iceberg	Wedge ⅛ of head	10	90	0.1

FOOD	SERVING SIZE	CALORIES	GRAMS	ENERGY DENSITY (cal/gr) Choose low values
Lettuce, Romaine	1 cup, chopped	8	55	0.2
Mushrooms, Button	1 cup, sliced or diced	17	70	0.2
Mushrooms, Shiitake	2 oz. dried	162	55	0.3
Onions	1 cup, chopped	60	160	0.4
Parsley	1 teaspoon, chopped	2	4	0.5
Pepper, Green Bell	1 cup, strips	27	100	0.3
Pepper, Red Bell	1 large or 1 cup, strips	27	100	0.3
Potato, White	2¾" × 4¼"	220	202	1.1
Potato, Sweet	5" × 2"	117	114	1.0
Potato, Baked (new white or sweet)	1 potato	145		0.7
Radishes, Red	10 small (1" diam.)	20	100	0.2
Spinach	1 cup, chopped, raw	6	30	0.2
Spinach	1 cup, cooked	41	180	0.2
Squash, Summer	1 cup, cubed	26	130	0.2
Squash, Winter	1 cup, baked	75	205	0.4
Tomato	2½" diam.	21	100	0.2
Turnip Greens	¼ lb.	34	115	0.3
Water Chestnuts	4 chestnuts	12	25	0.5
Yams	¼ lb.	133	115	1.2

FRUIT

FOOD	SERVING SIZE	CALORIES	GRAMS	ENERGY DENSITY
Apples	1 medium (2¾" diam.)	59	100	0.6
Applesauce, Unsweetened	½ cup	43	100	0.4

FOOD	SERVING SIZE	CALORIES	GRAMS	ENERGY DENSITY (cal/gr) Choose low values
Apricots	1 medium	19	40	0.5
Avocado	1 medium	360	170	2.1
Banana	1 medium	108	118	0.9
Blueberries	1 cup	81	140	0.6
Cantaloupe	½ medium	96	270	0.4
Cranberries	1 cup	49	100	0.5
Dates, Fresh or Dried	5	114	40	2.9
Figs, Raw	2 medium	74	100	0.7
Figs, Dry	1 fig	45	19	2.4
Grapefruit	½ medium	39	120	0.3
Grapes	1 cup	61	90	0.7
Lemon (peeled)	1 medium	24	85	0.3
Lime	1 medium	30	90	0.3
Nectarine	1 medium	33	70	0.5
Orange	1 medium	64	140	0.5
Papaya	⅓ medium	39	100	0.4
Peach	1 medium	42	100	0.4
Pear	1 small	82	135	0.6
Persimmon, Native	1 medium	60	50	1.2
Pineapple	1 cup, diced	76	155	0.5
Plums	2 medium	36	65	0.6
Raisins	2 tablespoons	54	18	3.0
Raspberries, Red	¾ cup	50	100	0.5
Strawberries	1 cup	50	150	0.3
Watermelon	1 cup, diced	52	160	0.3
Apple Juice	1 cup, bottled	116	248	0.5
Grape Juice	1 cup, bottled	154	248	0.6
Grapefruit Juice	1 cup, fresh squeezed	93	248	0.4
Prune Juice	1 cup, bottled	181	253	0.7

FOOD	SERVING SIZE	CALORIES	GRAMS	ENERGY DENSITY (cal/gr) Choose low values
Vegetable Juice	1 cup	46	240	0.2
Orange Juice	1 cup	111	248	0.5

LEGUMES

FOOD	SERVING SIZE	CALORIES	GRAMS	ENERGY DENSITY
Beans, Garbanzo	¼ cup	60	50	1.2
Beans, Green	1 cup	31	100	0.3
Beans, Lima	½ cup	71	100	0.7
Beans, Pinto	½ cup	86	100	0.9
Cowpeas	½ cup	92	70	1.3
Lentils, Brown	½ cup	116	100	1.2
Peas	1 cup	72	140	0.5
Soybeans (Mature)	¼ cup	77	50	1.5
Soybean Curd (Tofu)	1 piece (2½" × 1" × 2¾")	115	120	1.0
Split Peas	½ cup	115	100	1.2
Burger, Veggie, Boca	1 burger	110		
Chili, Vegetarian, Fat-Free	½ cup	80		

HEALTHY CARBS: WHOLE GRAINS

Cereals, Grains, Breads

FOOD	SERVING SIZE	CALORIES	GRAMS	ENERGY DENSITY
Amaranth	1 cup, cooked	182	80	2.3
Buckwheat	1 cup, cooked	194	100	1.9
Bulgur	1 cup, cooked	151	182	10.8
Couscous	1 cup, cooked	175	157	1.1
Millet	1 cup, cooked	207	174	1.2
Quinoa	1 cup, cooked	211	170	1.2
Cereal— Rolled Oats	1 cup	311	80	3.9
Cereal—Rye	1 cup	260	80	3.3

FOOD	SERVING SIZE	CALORIES	GRAMS	ENERGY DENSITY (cal/gr) Choose low values
Shredded Wheat	1 biscuit	90	25	3.6
Oat Bran	1 cup, cooked	88	219	0.4
Oatmeal	1 cup, cooked	145	123	1.2
Wheat Flakes	1 cup	100	30	3.3
Wheat Germ	1 tablespoon	21	6	3.5
Wheat Bran	½ cup	60	24	2.5
Bread, Rye (American)	1 slice	89	32	2.8
Bread, Pumpernickel	1 slice	80	32	2.5
Bread, Mixed Grain	1 slice	80	32	2.5
Bread, Oat Bran	1 slice	70	32	2.2
Bread, Pita, Whole Wheat	1 small pita	74	28	2.6
Crackers, Health Valley, Whole Wheat, Low-Fat	6 crackers	60		3.6
Crispbread, Wasa, Light Rye, Fat-Free	1 slice	25		3.6

Other Grains and Flours, Pasta

Barley, Pearl	1 cup, cooked	193	157	1.2
Cornmeal	¼ cup	300	30	10.0
Gluten Flour	1 cup	378	140	2.7
Rice, Brown, Short-grain	¼ cup	171	50	3.4
Rye Flour	1 cup sifted	357	100	3.6
Wheat Bran	1 tablespoon	13	6	2.2
Wheat Flour, Enriched	½ cup sifted	203	60	3.4
Wheat Flour, Whole	½ cup sifted	203	60	3.4

FOOD	SERVING SIZE	CALORIES	GRAMS	ENERGY DENSITY (cal/gr) Choose low values
Wild Rice	¼ cup	41	40	1.0
Noodles, Soba	1 cup, cooked	112	114	1.0
Macaroni, Whole Wheat	1 cup, cooked	173	140	1.2
Spaghetti, Whole Wheat	1 cup, cooked	173	140	1.2
Popcorn, Plain-popped	3 cups	97	24	4.0
Popcorn, Microwave, Weight Watchers, Smart Snackers	1 package	100	28	3.6

UNHEALTHY CARBS: BAKED GOODS AND SNACKS

FOOD	SERVING SIZE	CALORIES	GRAMS	ENERGY DENSITY
Bagel, Egg	1 bagel (3" diam.)	247	89	2.8
Bagel, Whole-grain	1 bagel (3" diam.)	226	89	2.5
Biscuit, Buttermilk (refrigerator)	1 biscuit	93	27	3.4
Bread, Italian	1 piece	54	20	2.7
Bread, Raisin	1 slice	71	26	2.7
Cake, Angel Food	1 piece, 1/12 of 12 oz. cake	73	28	2.6
Cake, Carrot (no frosting)	1 piece, 1/12 of 18 oz. cake	176	42	4.2
Cake, Chocolate (with frosting)	1 piece, 1/18 of 18-oz. cake	234	64	3.7
Cake, Pound, Fat-Free	1 slice (1 oz.)	80	28	2.9
Cake, Pound (made with butter)	1 slice (1 oz.)	110	28	3.9
Cheesecake	1 piece, ⅙ of 17-oz. cake	257	80	3.2

FOOD	SERVING SIZE	CALORIES	GRAMS	ENERGY DENSITY (cal/gr) Choose low values
Chips, Potato, "Lite"	1¼-oz. bag	166	35	4.7
Chips, Potato, Barbecue	1¼-oz. bag	174	35	5.0
Chips, Potato, Salted Plain	1-oz. bag	115	28	4.1
Chips, Tortilla, Plain	1 oz. (about 15 chips)	142	28	5.1
Cinnabon Caramel Pecanbon	1 (8 oz.)	890	224	4.0
Coffeecake, Cheese	1 piece, ⅙ of 16-oz. cake	257	76	3.4
Cookie, Chocolate Chip	1 soft type	69	15	4.6
Cookie, Fig Newton	1 cookie	55	16	3.4
Cookie, Nabisco Oreos	1 cookie	52	11	4.7
Cookie, Oatmeal	1 big cookie, 3″ x 4″	112	25	4.5
Cookie, Oatmeal, Fat-Free	1 big cookie, 3″ x 4″	92	28	3.3
Cookie, Sandwich (with chocolate creme filling)	1 cookie	47	10	4.7
Cookie, Sugar	1 cookie	71	15	4.7
Cornbread	1 piece (about 2 oz.)	173	65	2.7
Cracker, Ritz	2 crackers	78	16	4.9
Cracker, Saltines	1 large round	43	10	4.3
Cracker, Sandwich (with cheese filling)	1 sandwich cracker	34	7	4.9
Cracker, Wheat Thin	1 cracker	14	3	4.7
Croissant, Au Bon Pain, Almond	1 (5 oz.)	630	140	4.5

FOOD	SERVING SIZE	CALORIES	GRAMS	ENERGY DENSITY (cal/gr) Choose low values
Danish Pastry	1 pastry	265	71	3.7
Doughnut, Chocolate (cake type, sugared)	1 doughnut	250	60	4.2
Doughnut, Jelly	1 doughnut	289	85	3.4
English Muffin, Sourdough	1 muffin	133	57	2.3
English Muffin, Whole Wheat	1 muffin	134	66	2.0
Melba Toast	1 slice	19	4	4.8
Muffin, Au Bon Pain, Carrot Pecan	1 (5 oz.)	480	140	3.4
Muffin, Blueberry	1 muffin	196	71	2.8
Pie, Apple	1 slice, ⅛ of 9-inch pie	296	125	2.4
Pie, Blueberry	1 slice, ⅛ of 9-inch pie	290	125	2.3
Pie, Coconut Cream	1 slice, ⅙ of 7-inch pie	190	64	3.0
Pie, Lemon Meringue	1 slice, ⅙ of 7-inch pie	302	113	2.7
Pie, Pecan	1 slice, ⅙ of 7-inch pie	452	113	4.0
Popcorn, Cheese Flavor	1 cup	57	11	5.2
Popcorn, Oil-Popped	1 cup	55	11	5.0
Pretzels, Salted Plain	10 twists	228	60	3.8
Pretzels, Whole Wheat	2 oz.	205	56	3.7
Rice Cakes	2 cakes	68	18	3.8
Scone, Starbucks, Maple Nut	1 scone	570		
Strudel, Apple	1 piece	194	71	2.7

FOOD	SERVING SIZE	CALORIES	GRAMS	ENERGY DENSITY (cal/gr) Choose low values
Trail Mix (with chocolate chips)	1 oz.	137	28	4.9
Turnover, Pepperidge Farm, Apple	1 turnover	284	89	3.2
Waffle, Plain	1 waffle	88	28	3.1

PROTEIN

Eggs

Egg, White	1 medium	17	33	0.5
Egg, Whole	1 medium	77	50	1.5
Egg, Yolk	1 medium	59	16	3.7

Seaweed

Hijiki	⅛ cup	5	8	0.6
Kombu	⅛ cup	6	8	0.8
Nori	⅛ cup	6	8	0.8
Wakami	⅛ cup	5	8	0.6

Nuts & Seeds

Almonds	14 medium	98	28	3.5
Almond Butter	1 tablespoon	101	16	6.3
Brazil Nuts	1 nut	18	3	6.0
Cashews	14 large	162	28	5.8
Chestnuts, Fresh Roasted	2 large	50	35	1.4
Filberts (Hazelnuts)	10 nuts	88	14	6.3
Macadamia Nuts	11 nuts (1 oz.)	199	28	7.1
Peanuts, Dry Roasted	1 tablespoon chopped, or 15 whole	165	28	5.9
Peanut Butter	1 tablespoon	94	16	5.9

FOOD	SERVING SIZE	CALORIES	GRAMS	ENERGY DENSITY (cal/gr) Choose low values
Pecans	10 large	189	28	6.8
Walnuts	1 oz.	172	28	6.1
Pumpkin Seeds	⅛ cup	90	17	5.3
Sunflower Seeds	⅛ cup	102	18	5.7
Tahini	1 tablespoon	85	15	5.7

Fish

FOOD	SERVING SIZE	CALORIES	GRAMS	ENERGY DENSITY
Bass, Black Sea	3½ oz.	124	100	1.2
Bass, White Sea	3½ oz.	124	100	1.2
Catfish	3½ oz.	103	100	1.0
Clams	4 cherrystone	51	70	0.7
Cod	3½ oz.	105	100	1.1
Crab (steamed)	3½ oz.	97	100	1.0
Haddock	3½ oz.	112	100	1.1
Halibut	3½ oz.	140	100	1.4
Herring, Pacific	1 herring	100	50	2.0
Lobster	1 cup cubed	142	145	1.0
Mackerel, Atlantic	3½ oz.	262	100	2.6
Ocean Perch	3½ oz.	121	100	1.2
Oysters	medium, 2 selects	66	25	2.6
Perch, White	3½ oz.	121	100	1.2
Red Snapper	3½ oz.	128	100	1.3
Salmon, Atlantic	3½ oz.	206	100	2.1
Salmon, Atlantic (canned)	1 small can (6½ oz.)	283	185	1.5
Sardines, Pacific	3½ oz.	208	100	2.1
Sardines, Atlantic (canned)	3½ oz.	208	100	2.1
Scallop, Raw	1 large	22	25	0.9
Scallop (breaded and fried)	1 large	66	31	2.1
Shark	3½ oz.	130	100	1.3

FOOD	SERVING SIZE	CALORIES	GRAMS	ENERGY DENSITY (cal/gr) Choose low values
Shrimp (raw)	3½ oz.	99	100	1.0
Shrimp (cooked)	4 large	21	22	1.0
Sole	3½ oz.	117	100	1.2
Squid	3½ oz.	92	100	0.9
Swordfish	3½ oz.	155	100	1.6
Tuna (canned)	½ cup	213	115	1.9
Sushi, Salmon	4 small pieces on rice with nori wrapper	160	N/A	
Meat & Poultry				
Bacon, Regular	3 medium slices	109	20	5.5
Bacon, Canadian-style	2 slices	86	45	1.9
Beef, Flank Steak (no visible fat)	3 oz.	224	85	2.6
Beef, Ground (extra-lean)	3 oz.	218	85	2.6
Beef, Ground (lean)	3 oz.	231	85	2.7
Beef, Ground (regular)	3 oz.	245	85	2.9
Beef, Loin/Sirloin	3½ oz.	226	100	2.3
Beef, Porterhouse Steak (lean)	3 oz.	190	85	2.2
Beef, T-Bone Steak	3 oz.	262	85	3.1
Beef, Top Sirloin	3 oz.	228	85	2.7
Beef, Round	3½ oz.	265	100	2.7
Beef Liver	3 oz.	136	85	1.6
Buffalo	3 oz.	111	85	1.3
Calves' Liver	3½ oz.	165	100	1.7
Chicken, Dark Meat	3½ oz.	192	100	1.9

FOOD	SERVING SIZE	CALORIES	GRAMS	ENERGY DENSITY (cal/gr) Choose low values
Chicken, Light Meat	3½ oz.	153	100	1.5
Chicken, Drumstick (medium-size, with skin)	1	112	52	2.2
Chicken, Drumstick (medium-size, skinless)	1	75	44	1.7
Ham, Canned	3½ oz.	239	100	2.4
Cured Ham	3 oz.	140	85	1.7
Hamburger Meat	3½ oz.	235	100	2.4
Lamb (cubed for kabobs)	3 oz.	158	85	1.9
Lamb, Rib	3 oz.	305	85	3.6
Lamb, Sirloin	3 oz.	248	85	2.9
Pork Chop, Loin (bone-in)	3 oz.	205	83	2.5
Pork, Sirloin Roast (bone-in)	3 oz.	221	85	2.6
Rabbit, Domestic	3½ oz.	197	100	2.0
Turkey, Thigh (with skin)	1 thigh	492	314	1.6
Turkey, Light Meat	3½ oz.	157	100	1.6
Turkey, Dark Meat	3½ oz.	187	100	1.9
Veal, Breast (boneless)	3 oz.	226	85	2.7
Veal, Loin	3½ oz.	217	100	2.2

CALCIUM-RICH FOODS

Milk and Soy Milk Products

Buttermilk	1 cup	99	244	0.4
Low-Fat Milk (2%)	1 cup	102	244	0.4
Skim Milk	1 cup	85	244	0.4
Whole Milk	1 cup	159	244	0.7

FOOD	SERVING SIZE	CALORIES	GRAMS	ENERGY DENSITY (cal/gr) Choose low values
Sour Cream, Nonfat	1 tablespoon	31	14	2.2
Yogurt, Low-Fat, Plain	1 container (8 oz.)	231	240	1.0
Yogurt, Low-Fat (containing fruit)	1 container (8 oz.)	220	240	0.9
Yogurt, Nonfat, Plain	1 container (8 oz.)	100–120	240	·
Yogurt, Low-Fat, Plain	1 container (6 oz.)	170–180	168	
Yogurt, Nonfat, Plain	1 container (6 oz.)	80–100	168	
Yogurt, Whole Soy, Plain	1 container (8 oz.)	140	240	0.6

CHEESE

FOOD	SERVING SIZE	CALORIES	GRAMS	ENERGY DENSITY
American	1 slice (2¼″ square)	106	28	3.8
Blue Cheese	1″ cube	61	17	3.6
Camembert	1″ cube	50	17	2.9
Cheddar	1″ cube	114	28	4.1
Cottage (dry)	1 cup	85	200	0.4
Cottage (1% fat)	¼ cup	40	60	0.7
Cream Cheese	1 tablespoon	50	14	3.6
Cream Cheese, Fat-Free	1 tablespoon	13	14	0.9
Feta	1″ cube	44	17	2.6
Goat Cheese, Semisoft	1 oz.	100	28	3.6
Monterey Jack	1″ cube	64	17	3.8
Mozzarella, Part-Skim	1″ cube	72	28	2.6
Parmesan	1 tablespoon	22	12	1.8
Ricotta, Part-Skim	½ cup	171	124	1.4

FOOD	SERVING SIZE	CALORIES	GRAMS	ENERGY DENSITY (cal/gr) Choose low values
Soy Cheese	1 oz.	70	28	2.5
Soy Cheese, Fat-Free	1 oz.	40	28	1.4
Swiss	1" cube	56	15	3.7

Frozen Confections

Ice Cream, Low-Fat	½ cup	178	120	1.5
Ice Cream, Sugar-Free	½ cup	98	120	0.8
Ice Cream, Chocolate	½ cup	142	120	1.2
Ice Cream, Eskimo Pie	1 bar	166	50	3.3
Ice Cream, Häagen-Dazs	½ cup	280	120	2.3
Ice Cream, Ben & Jerry's	½ cup	275	120	2.3
Ice Cream, Cascadian Farm, Sorbet & Cream	½ cup	110	120	0.9
Ice Milk, Weight Watchers, Fat-Free	½ cup	82	120	0.7
Ice Milk, Healthy Choice	½ cup	124	120	1.0
Yogurt, Frozen	½ cup	115	120	1.0
Yogurt, Frozen, Stonyfield Farm	½ cup	125	120	1.0
Soy "Ice Cream," Turtle Mountain It's Delicious	½ cup	120	112	1.1
Rice Dream	½ cup	120	112	1.1
Tofutti	½ cup	215	112	1.9
Sorbet, Dole	½ cup	50	112	0.5

FOOD	SERVING SIZE	CALORIES	GRAMS	ENERGY DENSITY (cal/gr) Choose low values
Sorbet, Häagen-Dazs	½ cup	170	112	1.5

HEALTHY OILS

FOOD	SERVING SIZE	CALORIES	GRAMS	ENERGY DENSITY
Canola Oil	1 tablespoon	120	14	8.6
Flaxseed Oil	1 tablespoon	120	14	8.6
Mayonnaise, Light	1 tablespoon	35	14	2.5
Olive Oil	1 tablespoon	120	14	8.6
Rape Seed	1 tablespoon	120	14	8.6
Safflower Oil	1 tablespoon	120	14	8.6
Sesame Oil	1 tablespoon	120	14	8.6
Walnut Oil	1 tablespoon	120	14	8.6

UNHEALTHY OILS

FOOD	SERVING SIZE	CALORIES	GRAMS	ENERGY DENSITY
Butter, Salted	1 tablespoon	100	14	7.1
Margarine, Tub-Style, 48% Fat	1 tablespoon	50	14	3.6
Margarine, Parkay	1 tablespoon	70	14	5.0
Margarine, Trader Joe's	1 tablespoon	100	14	7.1
Margarine, Whipped Light	1 tablespoon	23	14	1.6
Mayonnaise, Regular	1 tablespoon	100	14	7.1
Mayonnaise, Reduced Fat	1 tablespoon	50	14	3.6
Mayonnaise, Fat-Free	1 tablespoon	10	14	0.7
Mayonnaise, Canola Harvest	1 tablespoon	100	14	7.1
Corn Oil	1 tablespoon	120	14	8.6

FOOD	SERVING SIZE	CALORIES	GRAMS	ENERGY DENSITY (cal/gr) Choose low values
MISCELLANEOUS				
Dressing, Hidden Valley, Fat-Free (all flavors)	2 tablespoons	30	28	1.1
Dressing, Kraft, Light (all flavors)	2 tablespoons	50–60	28	
Dressing, Kraft, Honey Dijon	2 tablespoons	100	28	3.6
Dressing, Kraft, Thousand Island Bacon	2 tablespoons	130	28	4.6
Dressing, Kraft, Cucumber Ranch	2 tablespoons	140	28	5.0
Dressing, Naturally Fresh, Blue Cheese	2 tablespoons	170	28	6.1
Dressing, Naturally Fresh, Poppyseed	2 tablespoons	140	28	5.0
Dressing, Newman's Own, Ranch	2 tablespoons	140	28	5.0
Dressing, Wishbone, Fat-Free (all flavors)	2 tablespoons	40	28	1.4
Dressing, Wishbone, Classic Caeser	2 tablespoons	110	28	3.9
Dressing, Wishbone, Deluxe French	2 tablespoons	120	28	4.3
Dressing, Wishbone, Ranch	2 tablespoons	160	28	5.7
Ketchup	1 tablespoon	15	15	1.0
Mustard	1 teaspoon	15	5	3.0
Salsa, Tomato	¼ cup	18	N/A	

FOOD	SERVING SIZE	CALORIES	GRAMS	ENERGY DENSITY (cal/gr) Choose low values
Yeast	1 tablespoon	14	5	2.8
Jell-O, Sugar-Free, Low-Calorie	½ cup	7	N/A	0.1
Gelatin Desserts, Non-Sugar-Free	½ cup	79	N/A	
Ice Pops	1 bar (1.8 fluid oz.)	37	N/A	
Orange Marmalade	1 tablespoon	49	N/A	

HEALTHY SNACKS

Soup

Soup, Miso with Noodles, Low-Fat	1 cup	130	240	0.5
Soup, Black Bean, Fat-Free	1 cup	100	240	0.4
Soup, Health Valley, Lentil	1 cup	130	240	0.5
Soup, Health Valley, Pasta Parmesan	1 cup	100	240	0.4
Soup, Health Valley, 14 Garden Vegetable	1 cup	80	240	0.3
Soup, Progresso, Manhattan Clam Chowder	1 cup	110	240	0.5

FAST FOODS

Biscuit, Egg & Sausage	1 biscuit	580	180	3.2
Biscuit, Egg & Bacon	1 biscuit	458	150	3.1
Burrito, with Beans & Cheese	1 large	377	196	1.9

FOOD	SERVING SIZE	CALORIES	GRAMS	ENERGY DENSITY *(cal/gr)* *Choose* *low values*
Burrito, with Beans, Cheese & Beef	1 large	331	203	1.9
Cheeseburger (large double patty plus condiments)	1 serving	704	258	1.6
Cheeseburger (large single patty plus condiments)	1 serving	562	219	2.7
Cheeseburger (regular double patty plus condiments)	1 serving	460	160	2.9
Chicken Fillet Sandwich	1 sandwich	515	182	2.8
Chicken Nuggets, Plain (breaded and fried)	1 serving	287	106	2.7
Chicken Nuggets, with Barbecue Sauce (breaded and fried)	1 serving	330	130	2.5
Chicken, Dark Meat (breaded and fried)	2 drumsticks	430	148	2.9
Chicken, White Meat (breaded and fried)	1 breast	494	163	3.0
Chimichanga, Beef & Cheese	1 serving	443	183	2.4
Cookie, Chocolate Chip	1 box	232	55	4.2
Croissant, Egg & Cheese	1 croissant	368	127	2.9
Danish Pastry, Cheese	1 serving	353	91	3.9

FOOD	SERVING SIZE	CALORIES	GRAMS	ENERGY DENSITY (cal/gr) Choose low values
Danish Pastry, Fruit	1 serving	335	94	3.6
Fish Sandwich (with tartar sauce)	1 sandwich	431	158	2.7
Fish Sandwich (with tartar sauce and cheese)	1 sandwich	523	183	2.9
French Toast (with butter)	2 slices	356	135	2.6
Hot Dog (on bun with chili)	1	296	114	2.6
Ice Cream Sundae, Chocolate	1 sundae	284	158	1.8
Nachos, with Cheese	6–8 nachos	345	113	3.1
Nachos, with Cheese, Beans, Beef & Chilis	6–8 nachos	568	255	2.2
Onion Rings	8–9 rings	275	83	3.3
Potato, Baked (with cheese)	1 potato	473	296	1.6
Potato, Baked (with sour cream)	1 potato	392	302	1.3
Potato Salad	⅓ cup	108	95	1.1
French Fries, McDonald's	small serving, 2.4 oz.	210	68	3.1
French Fries, McDonald's	super-size serving, 7.1 oz.	610	198	3.1
French Fries, Burger King	small serving, 2.6 oz.	230	72	3.2
French Fries, Wendy's	small serving, 3.2 oz.	270	88	3.1
French Fries, Carl's Jr.	one serving, 3.3 oz	290	90	3.2
French Fries, Jack in the Box	regular serving, 4 oz.	350	112	3.1

FOOD	SERVING SIZE	CALORIES	GRAMS	ENERGY DENSITY (cal/gr) Choose low values
Pizza, with Cheese and Sausage	1 3" slice	336	129	2.6
Pizza, with Cheese and Pepperoni	1 3" slice	442	154	2.9
Shake, McDonald's McFlurry	small, 12 oz.	610	336	1.8
Shake, McDonald's Triple Thick	small, 16 oz.	570	480	1.2
Shake, McDonald's McFlurry	large, 16 oz.	890	480	1.9
Shake, McDonald's Triple Thick	large, 32 oz.	1,140	896	1.3
Shake, Burger King, Old Fashioned	22 oz.	760	616	1.2
Submarine, Roast Beef	1 sandwich	410	216	1.9
Submarine, Tuna	1 sandwich	483	256	1.9
Taco	1 small	369	170	2.2
Taco Salad	1½ cups	279	198	1.4
Yogurt, Frozen, Vanilla	½ cup	114	72	1.6

8
Parenting the Longevity Diet Lifestyle

Any major lifestyle change that you initiate involves several stages. First, you start to believe in the evidence that the change you are considering has actually had the desired effect in other people who have made that change. Next, you cultivate the belief that it will work for you. You tell yourself, "*I really need/want to do this; I know it will help me*," draw up a plan, and then work systematically from point A to point B and beyond; or maybe you just jump right in and build your path as you move along. Perhaps you enlist the aid of a buddy, or join a support group, to help keep you on track.

Next comes the trial-and-error stage, when your faith in the evidence, your resolve, your experiences as compared with your original expectations and your actual progress, and your support system (if applicable) will be tested. Finally, you assess the gains or sacrifices of your decision and either stay on board with your program or shift gears, subtly or otherwise.

Andrew went through this process several times:

> I tried diet after diet—the usual fruitless search, and classic yo-yo weight loss/gain. Some diets worked briefly, some didn't work at all, but even when they worked, the weight all went back on eventually whenever I stopped or got bored with whatever dietary restrictions were involved. I've been doing CR seriously for about fourteen months now. I've lost about thirty pounds. And why did CR stick? I suppose my need for long-term weight control and good nutrition gave me the persistence to stick to it so that I could pursue my love of sports well into old age.

Andrew was convinced to begin the Longevity Diet by the scientific evidence for it, and the stories of others on the CR Society e-mail list. Or, as Andrew enthused,

> They're an amazing bunch of characters on the CR mailing list. This is the first time I've actually felt like I'm part of an exciting, real-time experiment with other real people who think and feel the same way I do. Long may we thrive!

How to Begin

Your Contract

Once you decide that you are ready to try the Longevity Diet, make a contract with yourself. (Well, let's back up. Once again: Talk to your physician first!) Writing things down will help you clarify why you want to do this, and how you plan to go about it. For example, Andrew wants to be healthy enough to run a marathon well into old age. For him, the Longevity Diet is a means toward something that he loves.

What does a contract look like? It could be something very formal, or akin to a letter you might send a good friend. How detailed you may wish it to be, is purely up you. Here's an example:

> From today onward and for at least the next ____ I choose to follow a longevity diet program that consists of selecting foods that nourish me. I will gradually eat fewer calories.
>
> Today I weigh ___. My goal will be to eat sensibly, not merely to reduce my weight, as I understand that too-fast weight loss may present a hardship to my body. I plan on losing _____ per week.
>
> I respect what happens under my skin and want to learn as much as I can about the Longevity Diet. I understand that this is "CR," not "FR," mere food restriction. It is a longevity diet only if I'm eating foods replete with nutrients, such as vegetables, fruits, and whole grains. A balanced diet is crucial for a successful experience.
>
> If I begin to doubt or have problems with my program, I will seek the advice of my health-care practioner and someone familiar with the Longevity Diet.
>
> I plan to live long enough to see (the next century, a solar eclipse, a few great-great grandchildren; you can be creative here).
>
> Signed and dated:

Set six months or longer as your trial period. It takes time for your taste buds to transform and for you to crave healthy foods, if you didn't before. Be patient. Anything really worth doing takes a while to master, particularly when it is something that is custom-fitted for you. Since you will design a program that best suits your lifestyle and food preferences, the road map to success is in your hands—although many others have traveled a similar path and will offer suggestions, ultimately your transition will be unique to you.

You may want to read your contract on a daily basis, or use it as a gauge to monitor your progress weekly.

Be prepared to have days when your particular emotional triggers or stressful events lead you to backslide into old habits. This is perfectly normal, and nothing to feel guilty about. Just try, at the beginning, to stick to your contract as best you can, resuming your healthful diet as soon as possible. You may want to buy or make a calendar and mark *G* for great days and *D* for difficult days. Note on the calendar what event challenged your resolve. Social issues? Work? Family? Then, knowing that you might be faced with another challenging event, prepare yourself mentally to handle that situation differently, to not use food as a solution to a circumstance that does not, at its core, even involve food. It could help to have a few sugar-free mints or your favorite tea on hand for emotional emergencies—a small, nondestructive yummy something going down your gullet may be all you need to feel better.

Learn

Every veteran CR practitioner recommends that you learn as much as you can about good nutrition and healthy foods. This is especially important if you *really* want to extend your life span and pursue a more regimented Longevity Diet program. Fulfilling the nutritional requirements of someone with a low body mass index is essential for good health, especially in regard to sufficient consumption of protein and calcium.

When we on the Longevity Diet reach for an apple, the first thing we think of is its great taste. But by now we also know that it is antioxidant rich, and that it contains a high level of a beneficial fiber, pectin. Before you make a financial investment, don't you research it? Isn't health your best investment? Read up on heart-healthy fats, antioxidant-rich foods, and phytonutrients, so that you, too, can appreciate what you eat not only as flavors and aromas, but as long-term sources of nutritional "dividends" for your body.

Strategize

Set small achievable goals, such as filling in the Daily Food Diary with every morsel of food for a week, consciously substituting a low-calorie, healthy food for a high-calorie or processed one. This activity by itself will put you in charge of minute-by-minute decisions that do not eliminate but merely exchange food, such as eating a banana instead of carrot cake, or having a cup of tea with a few almonds, rather than a bagel, to help you make it through the midmorning slump.

Prepare

Prepare psychologically as well as physically. The contract, a buddy system, and a few pertinent questions about your habits and history with food and diets should help you. Take honest stock of where you're at: your emotional state, your ability to commit to things, and your natural proclivities. Have you tried to lose weight before? Was it difficult? If it was, you may need to set strong boundaries. We will give you some suggestions. Even if you know that you easily adapt to self-selected routines, it will still benefit you to prepare by learning as much as you can about CR and nutrition, as you may be unconsciously carrying the program of other diets' incorrect information about foods and your body's use of them.

From an ancient Vedic text comes this pertinent idea:
Watch your thoughts; they become words.
Watch your words; they become actions.
Watch your actions; they become habits.

Find Support

This may be posting motivational notes on the refrigerator, calling a friend, or even a "cr-onversation"—an imaginary dialogue with your self about health and the Longevity Diet, whenever you need an ally. Imagine yourself vital, alert, healthy. April has a great sense of humor—read her "cr-onversation with Myself at 4:30 a.m.":

"Now, self, you know you have to eat your egg whites for breakfast before you leave for work."

"But I don't want to! It's four thirty in the morning and you know I don't like to eat breakfast!"

"I know you don't like to eat breakfast, but you barely ate anything yesterday because you stupidly ordered the dead fish after saying you wouldn't, took three bites of it, and decided to feed the rest to the cat. And it made you feel sick for the rest of the day. No more dead fish, self. But now you're low on energy, very low in protein, and you have a busy day ahead. You have to eat your egg whites."

"Can't I just skip breakfast and promise to eat something later, when I'm not feeling so, well, four thirty a.m.-ish?"

"Have you not understood anything that you've read in the last three months? Breakfast is important, and protein is even more important. If you don't eat your egg whites, which give you a 29-gram head start on your protein quota, you know you won't eat enough protein later to make up for it. Protein makes you strong! You want to live a long time and be healthy, not look like a waifish supermodel! If you don't eat your protein, you'll never be strong enough to live to 110, and you'll never get to be six feet tall."

"What if I eat a Dunkin' Donuts bagel instead? That's food. And I'm pretty sure that the Longevity Diet won't make me six feet tall, even if I do get enough protein."

"That's a big waste of calories for almost no nutrition! Remember, the last time you did that you were distinctly underwhelmed by the taste. You've grown out of such silliness, little self. You're right about the height thing, though. The Longevity Diet won't make you taller. I get confused. It's been a rough week."

"It's been a rough week. And yesterday was a bad eating day . . . FR, not CR, due to the unfortunate demise of our lunch. The cat sure liked the salmon."

"So are you going to eat those egg whites?"

"Okay, I'll eat my egg whites."

"How about a glass of skim milk with that? Remember, we're working on calcium."

"Don't push your luck."

Remember, the Longevity Diet is not "just another diet" nor is it, indeed, a weight-loss program. It is a quality-of-life program. It is not about deprivation or hunger. *You will, however, lose weight.* You should, therefore, savor, relish, and enjoy your life on the Longevity Diet. Think of everything you learn about nutrition and your unique metabolism as having a positive impact upon not only your body but your mind. Note that several comprehensive health programs, such as Dean Ornish's Life Choice and the Okinawa Program, specifically incorporate body-mind techniques to reinforce healthy choices. Your initial projection, day-by-day awareness, and growing appreciation of your improving behaviors are the fundamental building blocks to a successful lifestyle makeover.

As Andrew recommends,

From one who has been through [the Longevity Diet]— learn about your body, its care and maintenance—it's the only one you have, so learn to love it. . . . Be aware of the stressors that might make you want to lose confidence in yourself, especially if that leads to overeating. Work, love life, daily commute; we all have them. Know yourself, and trick yourself into ignoring them. There are many such tricks; taking a few deep breaths, a few motivational words. With practice you can rise above these issues. And to help gain insight and control, try a course in meditation. If nothing else, you'll enjoy the time out.

And April says,

My particular brand of the diet has evolved a lot over a short period of time. In the beginning, I was just cutting out most junk foods, eating less of what I had eaten before, and substituting salad for pasta and bagels. As I became more serious and went through a period of reading the CR Society Archives, I drastically changed the content of my diet and dropped my calorie levels. Throughout the process, I've had occasions when I've eaten more calories than usual, or eaten foods I now only rarely eat. This isn't "cheating" because the Longevity Diet is not a dictatorial diet in the normal sense . . . it's about eating as few calories as you can without eating less of other nutrients essential for health.

Monitoring the Longevity Diet Lifestyle

Are You a Warrior or an Explorer?

The Warrior's Code

If there is a bag of chips on the counter, can you eat just a few? Do you have a hard time choosing between salad and creamed soup as an appetizer? Then following the Longevity Diet will call upon your finest resources to remain strong in your resolve to have a healthier body! As in the first step in any twelve-step recovery program, you first need to admit that you may have felt powerless to resist (in this case) the call of the refrigerator, or perhaps of your stomach. That does not mean you will fail on the Longevity Diet; quite the contrary. Eating for longevity gets you to become proactive against your inner wimp, by becoming knowledgeable about nutrition and imposing some behavioral rules that will tell your belly who's boss. Along with these strengths, you need to develop the flexibility to roll with life's punches in ways that will not derail your nutritional wagon.

As discussed earlier, we all have emotional triggers or other externally motivated behavioral patterns that may undermine our goals for health and well-being. When you begin the Longevity Diet, those triggers and patterns will at first raise their volume, begging for your attention, *precisely* because you have become so aware of your desire not to hear them. While your office mates snack at their desks before lunch hour, or your kids tear into an aromatic pizza, your inner dialogue may nag that you, too, really deserve a little treat. Be prepared with a counteroffensive: "skillful willpower," not to consume *nothing*, but to rethink your definition of a "treat": nibble on something healthy—a small handful of dried apricots or almonds, an apple, a big bowl of low-fat soup that has its own yummy fragrance. A large mug of green tea or just a glass of water with a squirt of citrus might even do the trick, if your mouth and then your stomach are contented by simply a feeling of being filled.

If temptation really rules in your roost, then you may need to clean out your kitchen and remove the seductive foods that lure you to give in. Cultivate strong will and don't order or cook the kinds of things that cause you to overeat. Cook with portion sizes in mind, storing or freezing the foods in individual servings. If you bring a "doggy bag" of food home from a restaurant, remember that it constitutes a second meal, not a second serving as soon as you are home. If hunger strikes, reach for any and every kind of fruit or vegetable, preferably one that takes a while to peel or chew. Try setting aside twenty minutes on a weekend to prepare vegetable snacks and small servings of nuts as snacks for the coming week. Store them in sandwich-size plastic bags so you can see what's in them and easily carry them with you.

Think of yourself as a warrior facing down an enemy—not food per se, but a simple yet pernicious thing: poor eating habits. Gluttony, one of the seven deadly sins, will initially fight for its right to control you, but forewarned is forearmed: now that you know your intention is to eat more wisely, you already have an argument ready for those moments when a pineapple Danish waves at you from the deli counter as you wait for your whole-grain toast. You may sometimes lose a battle, but you are determined to win the war.

You need strong weapons to combat everyday minefields. One solution may be as simple as reciting to yourself an affirmation, a mantra. In the 1920s, a well-being movement had followers telling themselves each morning, "Every day, in every way, I am getting better and better." April shared with us her own jingle: "We are Dr. Walford's mice, we find a longer life quite nice." You can imagine how surprised and warm this made us feel! And it worked for her. Focusing on the positive, on every refusal to give in, being one step closer to your ultimate goal, will help to underscore that calorie restriction is *not* deprivation, but a honing down of your diet to the most healthful essentials.

Consider it a victory every time you stop yourself from reaching for a food your body does not even want, every time you recognize and tune out a trigger or external cue. After a while, you will automatically make the right choices, but as you begin the program you will need to consciously jog yourself into a state of nutritional awareness, one that reshapes your old, poor eating habits into good ones. Imagine, for instance, that you are having a dialogue with a sibling, your spouse, a mentor, or a Longevity Diet role model—with someone who cares about your well-being and who wants you to be around for a long, long time. Hear them say, as did April's "cr-onversation" partner, "Come on, does this food really nourish you? What about having some nice ____ instead?"

A genuine in-the-flesh buddy system may help immensely, too. Phone an empathetic friend or drop by a colleague at work, to keep a supportive person abreast of what successes and failures you've had. The CR Society and its various support groups are great resources. Many people have celebrated weight loss, been warned of possible nutrition deficiencies or haphazard dieting, and found role models through these virtual groups. As we mentioned earlier, Andrew found a lot more than support from an online group.

The Warrior's Code will help you to harness your will power by reallocating your food choices and dealing with behaviors that undermine your health. Because you are probably going to find this program an uphill climb, with many questions, we recommend that you eat fairly structured meals and keep a Daily Food Diary along with a valiantly honest Nutrition Tracker, for as long as it takes to feel your new eating habits are second nature with you.

After six months juggling her routines, April recorded in her blog:

> Now I'm making different choices. I don't always get it right, but I'm glad that, as the work pressure goes up, I'm sticking with my resolve. I feel so much better on a daily basis than I did before. It's unfortunate that most people throw their healthy habits (if they ever had any) out the window the second life becomes stressful. It is when you're stressed that you most need your healthy habits!

The Explorer's Trail

Were you excited by the first half of this book? If you were, then you are the kind of person who wants to digest all the information you can and make a conscientious decision on how best to proceed. You believe that the evidence indicates that the Longevity

Diet will be great for you, and accept that you will be fully in charge of how to go about implementing the diet. You already feel those creative juices flowing as you look forward to designing, coordinating, and navigating your way through our recommendations.

You already understand that it is all about wholesome food and fewer calories, and that the rest is just mix and match, according to what works for you. Some people, like Peter Voss, graze throughout the day. Others, like Lee Shurie, eat one main meal a day. Still others, like Lisa, juice-fast one day per week. Dean Pomerleau prepares and eats the same meal every day. Some, like Khurram Hashmi, weigh and record all their foods. April, on the other hand, went freestyle and just made conversational-in-tone entries online in a blog for her first six months.

Because you are already attuned to the mind-body connection, following the Longevity Diet may be easier for you than for the Warrior first learning to read his or her inner signals. In your case, use the Daily Food Diary to track not what causes you to eat, but how you feel while your body is using what you have consumed. We find, for example, that eating a light protein meal midday maintains even energy levels in the afternoon. Whole grains, veggies, nuts, dairy protein, in whatever combination you may enjoy eating at night, can constitute a large supper, as long as it is predominantly veggies. Remember, vegetables are filled with phytonutrients, and are low energy-dense and high in fiber. If you can feel energetic in the morning without eating a big breakfast, don't feel you need to eat one to start your day; Lisa does her yoga in the morning, with no breakfast before practice. And yet most nutritionists say that breakfast is the most important meal of the day. Brian has followed that dictate all his life, and the Longevity Diet hasn't changed that. Do what literally feels right for your body.

Since you are already of the mind-set to choose an apple over an apple turnover, you should be able to make the transition to a moderate Longevity Diet without needing to counteract detrimental eating habits. Peter Voss suggests, when you go shopping, to fill your cart with wholesome foods. Don't bring home anything you know you should not eat. No need to nix the snack food already on your shelves, it will be overwhelmed by your conscious substitution of healthy choices, and gradually you'll stop feeling any desire to replace an emptied unhealthy package with another of the same product.

Lee's Story

It was not the Longevity Diet that salvaged what could have been a difficult life for Lee. It was his own ingenuity and persistence. There is nothing that dramatic about the Longevity Diet lifestyle, no secrets, no special food combinations, just good common sense. Highly motivated and savvy as he was, Lee rescued himself from a potentially life-debilitating disease and serendipitously found that he was actually on CR. He then became an inspiration to many on the CR Society mailing lists.

> When I was in my mid-forties I was diagnosed as diabetic. The slow, miserable decline associated with long-term diabetes presented a grim future for me, and I vowed to somehow find a cure—or at least a management program that would permanently keep the disease at bay. Because the medical profession does not have such a cure, I was determined to find one myself.
>
> I spent the first year refining my diet and kept a daily journal of everything I ate, including quantities, time of day, calories, protein, carbs, fat, and fiber content. The journal

also records exercise, blood sugar level, weight, and notes about my mental and physical condition. The journal helped me to successfully design a program to normalize my blood sugar levels. I now don't need any medication. I followed a strict regimen for months and months, during which time I ate only low-glycemic-index foods and lost approximately 15 pounds. Unfortunately, the switch to low-glycemic foods and the weight loss was not sufficient to fully counteract the disease. My blood sugar levels improved approximately 5 percent, but there was still work to be done. The next item I worked on was exercise. This wasn't easy, because I have two young children, social obligations, and am president of my own company. But it was absolutely necessary! Unfortunately, the switch to a vigorous exercise program was not sufficient to fully counteract the disease. My blood sugar levels improved another 5 percent, there was still work to be done.

As I continued my diet regimen I found that I was naturally consuming far fewer calories than before. I realized how important it was to choose highly nutritious foods. After experimenting and adjusting, I ended up on a low-calorie, nutrient-dense diet. Later I learned there is a scientific basis for the Longevity Diet: the decades of research into CR. And that one benefit of CR appears to be the improvement in blood sugar levels that I had stumbled upon. As I researched CR and longevity further, I found that many of the biometric and quality-of-life improvements that I had experienced were associated with the CR dietary approach. I now follow the diet with my own modifications regarding meal timing. I believe each person on this diet must tailor their own eating plan and schedule, and follow what works

in their body and with their lifestyle. I am quite active ath-
letically and often go all day at high energy levels, while
those who've eaten breakfast and lunch or energy snacks fall
behind. This routine works well for me, with my lifestyle,
and you will see from the graph that it has stabilized my
blood sugar levels dramatically

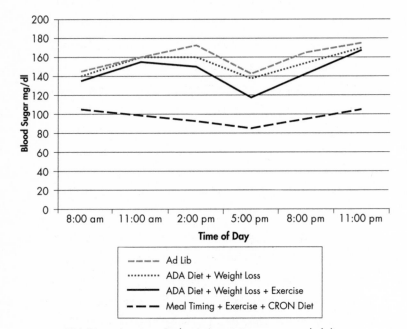

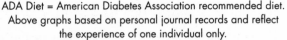

ADA Diet = American Diabetes Association recommended diet.
Above graphs based on personal journal records and reflect
the experience of one individual only.
Normal fasting blood glucose levels are typically defined as 80–100.
Prediabetes diagnosis begins at 126, and full diabetes is 145 or above.

I don't eat until 6:00 p.m., when I have a large salad with
quite a variety of goodies. With a foundation of fresh green
and cruciferous vegetables, tomatoes, and onions, I access-
orize it from day to day depending on the ingredients I have
available. If it is to be my only meal, then I may add an ounce
of low-fat mozzarella cheese, an ounce or two of leftover

baked chicken breast, 1 hard-boiled egg, and 8 or 10 nuts (mixture of almonds, cashews, and hazelnuts). The dressing is a homemade balsamic vinaigrette with extra-virgin olive oil. I often add a couple tablespoons of fresh salsa to spice things up, and sometimes a bit of prepared horseradish. At times, I'll alternate with 3 ounces of chicken breast, a 2-egg omelet, 1 ounce of low-fat-mozzarella cheese, or 3 ounces of fish (preferably sashimi). Note there are *no* breads, pastas, or grain/flour products whatsoever in my diet. Fruit is an occasional treat but not a staple. If you look at the USDA food guide pyramid, I've completely wiped out the bottom row. I never ever consume sugars or sweetened drinks—other than an occasional diet soft drink. I do make use of Splenda in my salad dressing—or if I need an occasional beverage sweetener. For me, this regimen is very easy to maintain. It fits with my lifestyle and my natural hunger patterns. Now I seldom get hungry during the day, even when I'm involved in strenuous sports activities. Prior to CR I ate the traditional three hearty meals a day plus snacks, but was nevertheless *always* desperately hungry. What I do advocate is to keep a journal when you experiment with new foods or eating patterns. This way you can learn exactly what works for *you*, regardless of the confusing and often incorrect literature and advice floating around on the subject of nutrition.

Are You a Calorie Counter or a Weight Watcher?

Other Approaches to Monitoring the Lifestyle Changeover
In the process of writing this book, we realized that some people like to improvise and others prefer to have a structured game plan. Both styles are effective, as long as you stick with the program. Whether you like to count calories or not is less important than

eating healthy foods and very gradually eating less of them, which will reduce your weight.

After a week or two of watching what you eat and filling your plate with ample amounts of colorful and whole, rather than processed, foods, the simplest way to begin the next phase of the Longevity Diet is to watch your weight. You don't need to be obsessive about weighing yourself, especially if you don't feel that you need to be on an extreme version of the Longevity Diet. Weighing yourself once or twice a week might suffice. There will be daily fluctuations in your weight, of course, but these won't matter at the beginning, especially if you're not radically restricting your caloric intake.

The ratio of protein to carbohydrates or fat is not as relevant as eating healthy foods and eating fewer calories. You don't need to eat smaller volumes of food. It depends on what kind of foods you choose to indulge in. If you prefer foods with low energy density, then your plate will be piled high with vegetables and whole grains, and topped with a smaller portion of protein. If you prefer a higher percentage of protein in your diet, then you will need to serve smaller portions. Both methods are health conscious; both work. You can decide which method *you* like.

Then, settle in for a few years of *very gradual* weight loss. This is not a deprivation diet. You should not have to go out and buy a new wardrobe in a few months. Losing weight quickly is counterproductive and will stress your body physiologically, possibly releasing toxins into the blood that were stored in fatty tissue. A life-extension diet is really a life maintenance diet, and hence not a reducing "diet" at all.

JW's Story—A Calorie Counter

JW's high blood pressure story attests to the dictate that calories count. When we first read about his initial days on the Longevity

Diet, we weren't sure we could use the details of his experiences. White rice? For the short run, JW's diet worked quickly and effectively to lower his blood pressure. He then conscientiously designed a wholesome diet. But it really demonstrates that it is the calories that will launch *your* healing journey as well.

In 2000 I was coerced into beginning CR. I depended on my beta-blockers and calcium channel-blockers to hold hypertension at bay. And I could not see my toes. . . . I woke up one morning disgusted with the ineptitude of doctors and nutritionists and decided to eat nothing. That quickly migrated to eating something "bland," so I opted for steamed rice, fat-free milk, and sugar. My blood pressure started dropping that day. At lunch I ate rice, strawberries, and fat-free milk. By suppertime, my BP was low enough I could skip the evening beta-blocker. This rice-based, low-sodium, low-protein diet continued for several weeks. My wife also went on this diet.

We had a diet that worked and I wasn't hungry. At about two months into the diet, my wife asked if that was all *we* were ever going to eat. She had gone from 185 to a beautiful 150. We started adding steamed veggies one at a time to test for allergies. I found I could eat almost any veggie steamed, and almost any fruit. We were lacto-vegetarian. I once said I would eat no meat forever, but since then I found I could eat a little meat as long as I did it without using salt. I leave off flavoring on veggies as well, so I can taste the true veggie taste. But my diet remains 95 percent lacto-veggie with a little fish, usually shellfish. Beef and pork are rare. Turkey, maybe once per year; chicken breast salad, maybe six times per year. Most pork, chicken, and turkey today is soaked in salt.

My weight didn't fall that much at first, it took about six weeks to drop down to 172 pounds from 206 pounds. At my roundest I weighed 234 pounds and it took me six years to work it down and up and down to 206 pounds. But rather than my new slender frame, my low blood pressure is what kept me on CR; and the looks for my wife. She's sixty-seven and looks maybe fifty years old. The effect was overwhelming for me. Practically all my wife's family have now lost weight and we have not pressured them at all. All are older than we are. Her bro-in-law is down from about 260 to maybe 190 now.

I developed a spreadsheet to keep track of foods I ate so that I could correlate it with blood pressure. I wrote a Basic program to massage the USDA database into a spreadsheet. That tool is basic to knowing what and how many calories I eat. Now I can judge the calories by eyeball. I now weigh 172.5 to 177.5. A key point I think is to cycle the weight up maybe five pounds, then down seven pounds, to maintain control. I plan to control it downward as I get older, maybe 165 next year, scaling down to 125 at age 100.

Peter Voss's Story—A Weight Watcher

Peter Voss is one of our longtime CR Society members. He and his partner, marathon runner Louise, frequently visited the late Dr. Roy Walford at his Venice Beach studio in California to discuss the Longevity Diet, as well as more "out there" futuristic topics like cryonics. Peter has perhaps the most flexible and well-adjusted attitude of any longtime practitioner of the Longevity Diet. Once you are well established with a routine that works for you, he says, "Most important, if CR becomes difficult, or if it makes you unhappy, relax and eat a little more!" Perhaps Peter's success can be attributed to his motto: "Rationality, give me the strength to change the things I can, the serenity to accept those that I can't, and the wisdom to know the difference."

When I started CR in 1997, I weighed 155 pounds. Now, seven years into this lifestyle, I have hit my cruise control and, with less than 5 percent body fat I don't think that I want to lose any more weight! The 1,800 to 1,850 calories a day I need to maintain my weight satisfies me; I feel strong and don't suffer from the frequent colds I used to before starting CR. Hunger was a problem in the beginning (I restricted fairly rapidly—more than I would recommend), but now I manage fine (it almost seems that my stomach has shrunk)! At first, I regularly monitored, recorded, and analyzed *all* the food I would eat for periods of about four weeks, and then go for two to three months without monitoring (other than my morning weight); but with the same eating habits. I lost weight slowly, not more than one pound per month. My blood pressure declined over the first two years to around 105/70.

I very gradually, over several years, cut back the serving sizes of high-calorie ingredients. For example, from one-half slice of full-fat cheese per cracker I cut back to one-eighth slice low-fat cheese, and I would use one tablespoon of salad dressing rather than two. Strangely, I've found that my taste buds adjusted and food seems even tastier now. I'm now able to discern more subtle textures and flavors.

I am a grazer, so many small meals savored throughout the day helped me maintain my energy. I have lots of desirable food readily available, with fruit on my countertop and veggies in the fridge. Green, black, and rooibos tea along with lots of water help keep me hydrated and full.

This is just background to the main point that I hardly ever cook, buy virtually all my food at the local supermarket chain store, and go out to eat frequently (I order with care: both what I select and changes I request. Minor adjustments can make a huge nutritional difference). I love strawberries, broccoli, spinach—veggies and more veggies, often with pasta sauce—salmon, chicken breast, almonds, steel-cut oats, yogurt (including frozen), hot chocolate (diet), and nonfat crackers with a little peanut butter and banana. I really love the food I now eat, and miss it when I can't get it.

Other Techniques for the Longevity Diet

Fasting

There have been many discussions amongst our group regarding the benefits and efficacy of fasting. A true fast consists of consuming only water. This strict, and potentially therapeutic, approach to ameliorating some disease warrants further research, and is beyond the scope of this book.

However, less stringent definitions of fasting are plentiful. Lisa abstains from food one day a week, drinking plenty of water and twelve ounces of diluted fruit or vegetable juice. While this is technically not a fast, it does shear 1,000 calories off of her weekly average, and gives her a day of rest from food anticipation, food prep, food consumption, cleanup, and digestion. These are her most productive days. Not only does Lisa ingest less food on her fasting days but food consumes less of her time that she can then funnel into other activities.

Fasting can be mentally strengthening as well as an easy way to cut calories. If you choose this strategy, we suggest that you pursue short fasts—do not fast for more than one or two days at a time—and drink plenty of fluids. If you have a serious health problem do not attempt to fast unless you are under the care of a physician. This includes diabetics and anyone taking prescription medicines.

10

The Longevity Diet and Exercise

While exercise, in and of itself, does not slow the aging process, for many people it can be an important element in a successful longevity program.

Aging and Cells

Do you run, pedal, swim, lift weights, or do yoga or tai chi? The truth is, although such activities will add life to your years, they will not necessarily add years to your life. Exercise can mitigate the effects of an unhealthy lifestyle: it can lower blood pressure, slow down or reverse arteriosclerosis, lower cholesterol, improve insulin metabolism, maintain and improve bone density, release endorphins, and reduce stress. However, while exercise helps extend the average life span of groups studied, virtually no studies have proven that such regimens improve the maximum life span of any species studied. That is, only the Longevity Diet will slow the aging process itself.

In 2000, calorie-restricted sedentary mice were compared with non-CR sedentary mice that could eat as much as they wanted, with CR mice who exercised, and with non-CR mice that exercised but could eat as much as they wanted. As expected, the non-CR sedentary mice became heavy, developed various cancers, diabetes, and grayed more quickly. Surprisingly, the CR mice that did not exercise looked like the non-CR mice that exercised and ate as much as they wanted—except that the CR mice that didn't exercise lived even longer![1]

More recent studies have attempted to identify the biological mechanisms through which CR and/or exercise improves cardiac function,[2] reduces inflammation,[3] inhibits neurodegeneration of the brain, and helps prevent breast cancer. The Diabetes Foundation, the American Heart Association, and the National Institutes of Health, among many other groups, are seeking to understand the molecular changes that appear to trigger such systemic beneficial results. But the studies point to a more complex story, with advances and retreats on both sides of the CR vs. exercise discussion.

For instance, a randomized, fully controlled study[4] out of Baton Rouge sought to measure the effects of six months of calorie restriction, with and without exercise, in overweight, non-obese men and women. At the end of the study period, the exercise and calorie-restricted groups were equally effective in reducing both weight and fat.

Lifelong, committed, long-distance runners generally don't die young. But they don't live extraordinarily long lives, either. Aerobic exercise is great for you. We all know that it reduces your odds of getting many of the diseases associated with aging. But it doesn't slow the aging process itself. Even if your goal of reduced risk of heart disease, type 2 diabetes, stroke, and other diseases of aging is achieved via the Longevity Diet, and not aerobic exercise, aerobic exercise will still make you feel good. It reduces the deleterious effects of stress, can help stave of depression, and can be a lot of fun!

Aerobics: Good for the Heart and Brain

If you're not on a rigorous Longevity Diet program, the traditional benefits of aerobic exercise are very much worth keeping in mind.

The American College of Sport's Medicine defines *aerobic exercise* as "any activity that uses large muscle groups, can be maintained continuously, and is rhythmic in nature." *Aerobic fitness* refers to your body's ability to get oxygen to your muscles. When your heart is strong, more oxygen-rich blood is pumped with each heartbeat. When you are not aerobically fit, your heart must beat faster and work harder to provide the oxygen required for any physical exertion. Hence, people who are not in good shape get out of breath quickly. Just like your biceps, the heart is a muscle, and it will respond and reward you when you work out diligently over a period of time.

Aerobic exercise, as with CR, also improves the brain's agility, that is, your ability to problem solve and reason things out. The brain, just like your muscles and organs, needs oxygen. With age, the oxidative decline throughout the body also largely affects front-brain activities. With our rapidly changing world, lifelong learning is essential, and you will need an agile mind. Brain health is best maintained by a rigorous Longevity Diet program. But for those not on a rigorous diet, evidence is pouring in that regular exercise maintains brain health. Researchers at the University of Illinois at Urbana–Champaign have shown that those who are fit perform significantly better on tests of cognitive function.[5]

Brisk walking, running, swimming, cycling, cross-country skiing, dancing, rollerblading, and stair climbing are a few common forms of an aerobic workout. If you are new to aerobic exercise, build up to twenty minutes gradually. Familiar theme? As with easing into the Longevity Diet, moderation will help trigger the body's adaptive process more effectively than the compulsive "new lease on life" that often sabotages a true lifestyle change. In addition, if you push too hard in the beginning you may get frustrated and strain muscles. Begin with brisk walking, a treadmill, or whatever is convenient, until you are a little short of breath, and slowly lengthen your sessions. If you begin to feel too comfortable while working out, this is a sign that you need to increase the relative difficulty of your regimen. For example, if walking one mile in twenty minutes has become easy, up your pace to cut the time to fifteen minutes. You need to feel your body reaching toward its goal, for the exercise to have an effect. Being slightly winded is good: it indicates that you are engaging your body's vital systems enough to build stamina and improve fitness, but not so much as to wear yourself out.

The effect of exercise is cumulative. If you have been aerobically active all your life, the cardiac benefits are greater than if you begin later on. However, some benefits depend on repeated and regular exercise. Increased sensitivity to insulin, for instance, declines only a few days after you stop exercising. If you are ill or injured, ease back into a lighter exercise routine as soon as you can; and get into the habit of raising a sweat at least briefly on a lazy day.

Resist overdoing it. Much more than thrice-weekly twenty-minute aerobic sets may run contrary to optimal health. The demands imposed on the body by, for example, a marathon run can cause damaging oxidative stress (free radical production) that is counterproductive to its otherwise favorable effects on your heart. Be mindful not to adopt an exercise regimen that exhausts your energy rather than enhances it. Learn to distinguish between stretching and strengthening your body, and straining it. Addictive zeal may lead to a sport therapy clinic, arthritic knees, or worse.

LOUISE

Louise Gold has been running for thirty years and has participated in thirty-one marathons, often placing or winning her age group. She applies the principals of the Longevity Diet and CR into her lifestyle to support her love for the run.

Louise said: I have always been interested in the relationship between great athletic ability and nutrition. I was a marathon runner prior to starting CR, and I ate enough to make sure that I had enough energy to maintain my stamina, not necessarily for longevity benefits. But as I learned how CR affects health and longevity, I began fine-tuning my diet.

Now I practice yoga four to five times a week. I still run, I do a long run every Sunday, ten to fourteen miles on hilly terrain, and two or three days a week I will run three to four miles.

Weight-Bearing Exercises and Resistance Training: Good for the Bones

Weight-bearing exercise and resistance training are important for everyone, even those on more rigorous versions of CR.

The disease **osteoporosis,** or "porous bones," currently affects 8 million women and 2 million men, with an additional 34 million at risk for low bone density and fractured hips, wrists, or vertebrae. The statistics are scary; in people over the age of fifty, 1 in 2 women and 1 in 4 men will experience some osteoporosis-related fracture in their remaining lifetime. Additional risk factors include being thin, having a small frame, low testosterone levels in men, long-term treatment with corticosteroids, lack of exercise, and a low calcium intake (common with a vegan or milk-free diet). In particular, Caucasian menopausal women undergo hormonal changes that can weaken their bones.

Your bones are living tissues, constantly being renewed. As a normal part of its life cycle, old bone is broken down and re-absorbed into the body and new bone is formed. This process is called *remodeling*. When you are about thirty years of age, your body will begin to absorb bone mass at a rate that outpaces your its ability to generate new bone. This process is normal, whether you drank your milk as a child or not. The good news is: Bones do respond to outside stimuli, such as weight-bearing exercise or resistance training. In fact, if you x-ray the arm of a tennis player, you will see that the bones in the playing arm are thicker and denser than the bones in the other arm.

An exercise routine for the bones should include weight-bearing and resistance-training exercises.

Weight-Bearing Exercise

The term *weight-bearing exercise* is quite literal: an activity in which you bear weight and resist gravity. This does not mean you need to lift weights. In such exercises, you are in fact carrying your *own* weight. Examples of weight-bearing exercises are walking, running, and stair climbing. On the other hand, swimming (in which water supports your weight) and bicycling (in which the bicycle itself does) may be among your aerobic favorites and are excellent for the heart, but they will not benefit your bones. So whether you choose a health spa with its treadmills and NordicTrack machines, or twenty minutes jogging outdoors in the fresh air and sunshine, your bones will bear testimony to your efforts and reward you with good density. Keep in mind that, while weight-bearing activities will strengthen the bones to the legs and hips, they are not as effective on the upper body, unless you pursue such activities as rock climbing or ball-hitting sports that create an interplay between your body's weight and the muscles of your arms.

Resistance Training

Resistance training, also known as *bone-loading exercise,* stresses the bones in another way, by exerting the pressure of muscular contraction. As your muscles contract and extend, the tendons that connect muscle to bone pull on the bone, and this pressure stimulates the tissues in the bones themselves. Hence, in a well-designed sequence, you would use all the major muscle groups in your arms, legs, and torso to reinforce a balance to the flexor and extensor muscles and an even distribution of pressure on the bones.

> Some in our CR community have reported a loss of bone density disproportionate to their age. Whether you jog, treadmill, lift weights, or practice yoga, bone loading exercise is probably an important addition for serious practitioners of the Longevity Diet.

Proper technique, good posture, and sequencing are vital for safety and to target specific muscles and bones. In sequencing a routine, it is important to warm up the body sufficiently before you start and to proceed through the exercises in the correct order, so find an instructor, a class, a video, or a good book on the subject before you begin. Health clubs are a valuable resource for equipment and expertise. Usually they have posters with safety tips and recommendations for using their weights and machines hanging on the walls, and they should have staff on hand to advise you on posture and technique. For convenience, various kinds of weights may also be purchased to be used at home.

Getting Started

For your arms, shoulders, and upper back, select a weight that you can lift easily eight times and practice repetitions until the muscle fatigues after ten to twelve cycles. Increase the weight by no more than 10 percent after you can comfortably practice with your beginning weights. Too much weight will increase any risk of injury, so take your time. Research indicates that *a single set* of a dozen repetitions with the proper weight is just as effective for bone mass as three sets. Again, less, when done properly, is more.

Do not underestimate the importance of good posture. Lift and lower weights slowly, this will minimize any risk of injury and maximize the strength building and bone-loading effects. Sore muscles or a little stiffness the day after exercise is normal, but throbbing or searing pain is a sign of nerve impingement or aggravation to tendon, ligament, muscle, or joint. With a brief period of complete rest, the body will usually recover on its own. When you do resume your routine, reduce the amount of weight you lift and build back with fewer repetitions. If pain persists or interrupts your sleep, see a doctor. And be patient—strength training is a slow process. Begin slowly and gradually build up a longer, more heavily weighted practice over a period of several months.

Exercise and Calories

Regular exercise not only burns calories, it also builds lean muscle mass and thus raises the *resting metabolic rate* (RMR). How? Remember that metabolism is the process that extracts and utilizes energy from food. Your resting metabolic rate is the amount of energy required to maintain your most basic body functions, such as respiration and cell repair. The minimum number of calories you need to eat while you are doing *absolutely nothing* is your resting metabolic rate. This accounts for approximately 70 percent of the energy you use every day. Lean muscle requires more energy (much like how a high-performance car engine prefers supreme gasoline) and burns more calories than fat, even at rest. If your primary goal is weight loss, this is particularly important.

Q. So if I am a power lifter or run daily and am on the Longevity Diet, should I eat more?

If you are physically fit and thin, you will have a greater percentage of lean muscle and will have a higher resting metabolic rate, and hence you may need to eat more calories than a heavier person who does not exercise. It is precisely for this reason that too much exercise is counterproductive to the Longevity Diet. Regardless of your exercise routine, your current weight, and your daily caloric intake, remember that your overall weight and moderation in all CR-related physical activities are key to good health.

Louise Gold explained it this way to us: Many people think that by running so much you can eat more calories, but you still have to keep your calories down. What people don't talk about is that much as CR decreases your metabolism, running does the same thing. Most runners who have run for many years know that running does not require much effort, once you get to the skill level that professionals have, the calorie needs go down and the body processes its energy reserves more efficiently.

Yoga: The New Wave

Yoga is good for more than just your peace of mind!

While the roots of yoga lie in the ancient application of body-mind practices to relieve suffering and to elevate consciousness, there are many relevant similarities between yoga and the Longevity Diet. These verses from the *Hatha Yoga Pradipika* were written in the fifteenth century:

> *Moderate diet means pleasant, sweet food, leaving free one fourth of the stomach.* 1.58
> *When the breath wanders, the mind also is unsteady. But when the breath is calmed, the mind too will be still, and the yogi achieves long life. Therefore, one should learn to control the breath.* 5.2[6]

Today yoga practices are frequently associated with stress reduction, flexibility, and breath awareness. But perhaps there is not that much difference between our quest for health and happiness with calorie restriction as there was for the yogis of the Middle Ages. When we recognize the continuum among the body (what we eat), the mind (attitudes, what we think), and the breath (breath awareness, the bridge between anxiety and relaxation), we can better address health comprehensively.

Lisa began teaching yoga in the early 1980s.

"When I first started teaching, if I told people that I taught yoga, they would say: 'Oh, you wave incense and chant.' 'Not exactly,' I would reply. Now, people say: 'Oh, you mean that I will sweat and get a good workout.' 'Not exactly,' I now reply."

Our contemporary understanding of yoga is largely based on reports in the mass media. Christine Turlington appeared on the cover of *Time* magazine in 2001 in a feature article titled, "The Science of Yoga: Millions of Americans are Discovering this Ancient Exercise—Here's the Skinny on Why It Makes You Feel So Good." That was the beginning of yoga as a modern-day industry. In 2005, *Time* again featured a cover story: "Lose That Spare Tire!

A Special Report on How to Get Fitter, Faster." Yoga was listed as a form of weekly exercise enjoyed along with riding a bike, hiking, and golfing. Yoga included as a statistic in *Time* magazine! This publicity shows us that yoga is now a commercially acceptable part of an integrated body-mind practice in any health program.

In 1994, the federal government formed the National Center for Complementary and Alternative Medicine (CAM) to monitor and assess the efficacy of various health modalities, practices, and products that are not generally considered part of regular medicine. While there are many CAM therapies—acupuncture, chiropractic, and massage, which are based on working with a practitioner, as well as deep breathing exercises, guided imagery, and tai chi—yoga is becoming particularly prominent. Natural products top the chart, followed by deep breathing, meditation, chiropractic and osteopaths, massage, yoga, diet-based therapies (like the Longevity Diet), progressive relaxation, and guided imagery.

With roughly 40 percent of adults seeking CAM therapies, medical professionals want to know statistically how well these practices work. Scientific studies point to the healing benefits of yoga as a complementary therapy for many conditions, including hypertension, chronic bronchitis, diabetes, arthritis, low back pain, headache, and sleep disorders.[7] According to a survey conducted by the Iyengar Yoga National Association of the United States, back pain, allergies, joint and muscle problems, depression, headaches, and anxiety are the main reasons people begin a yoga practice. The National Institutes of Health funded two randomized control studies on low back pain relief through yoga practice, both recommending yoga as a viable means to alleviate low back pain.[8] People suffering from depression,[9] insomnia,[10] osteoarthritis,[11] and many other conditions are improving through a yoga practice.

The restorative mechanisms within the body that particular poses seem to trigger are not well understood and depend on many variables, including the type of yoga practiced. Just as you would go to different specialists for low back pain and diabetes, the therapeutic application of yoga is a sophisticated and burgeoning discipline. In spite of the diversity of yoga styles, we can agree that stress reduction, breath control, flexibility, and concentration or mindfulness are helpful for any condition, either as a wellness tune-up or for remedial purposes. As with the Longevity program, you have to find what is appropriate for you!

How Does Yoga Differ from Other Forms of Exercise?

Breath and body awareness are integral to a yoga practice; in fact, they are the keystone that identifies yoga as distinct from other forms of exercise. You can sensitize yourself to the many messages speaking through your muscles, skin, and nervous system through yoga. Some of these messages are obvious; when you slouch, the upper back muscles tighten, you compress your diaphragm, and bear down on the abdomen. But some messages are much more subtle, yet very potent. Chronic physical tension is expressed in many ways. For example, squeezing your forehead, either because of poor vision or out of habit, or tightening your throat and lips add up and cheat you of focus, energy, and composure. The physical awareness encouraged through yoga helps you to recognize where you need to let go.

Deep breathing is the second most commonly practiced CAM therapy and the most popular do-it-yourself natural relaxation technique. Yoga practices are built around quieting and deepening the breath while cultivating a respect for the effect that the breath has on both the body and the mind. Mr. B. K. S. Iyengar, a yoga legend at ninety-two years of age and still going strong, states, "As leaves move with the wind, your mind moves with your breath."

Breath awareness can become a buffer and a bridge between you and your reactive emotions. And it is always available, every breath you take! It is ready to pick you up if you are drowsy or quiet you down if you are upset. The axiom "think before you speak" can better be expressed by "take a deep breath and exhale." It only takes a split second to catch the difference between your immediate knee-jerk reaction and a mature response in any situation. Yoga practice teaches you to watch the breath in every moment, and how to use the breath effectively to maintain your mental poise. Yoga instructors will guide you to observe when you are "over-efforting" or breathing incorrectly. In addition, by encouraging good posture and by stretching the auxiliary breathing muscles, yoga helps you breathe more easily.

Yoga will help you stretch your hamstrings, relieve your backache, and enable you to sleep better. It may deepen your appreciation for life by cultivating sensitivity and respect for your body. Yoga can be socializing: It may plug you into a community that supports wellness and get you in touch with healthy lifestyles. And over time, yoga can change the shape of your body, just like any good exercise program.

By comparison, a good weight-training program will incorporate form and alignment into how you lift, but it typically targets particular muscles in isolation from the body as a whole. Yoga poses integrate the entire body in a wide range of motion, lateral stretches, back strengtheners, loosening the hips and shoulder muscles; twists to relieve the small deep muscles that run alongside your spine; inverted poses that can passively increase cardiac output,[12] and restorative poses. In a good class, every major body part will be addressed to strengthen, stretch, and increase the range of motion in the joints. One caveat: Most kinds of yoga are not aerobic by nature, although there are some very athletic styles.

Yoga postures can also "stress" bone while stretching muscles, presumably the perfect combination. In fact, certain styles of yoga qualify as both weight-bearing and resistance training, while stretching out your muscles and lubricating all your joints to boot. A yoga method where you stay in the posture for at least a minute, and in particular standing postures and inversions (such as the "Downward Facing Dog" pose), offer the most in weight-bearing and bone-loading benefits.

Yoga is largely an isotonic form of exercise, wherein you strengthen muscle by using controlled movement and the resistance of the muscles themselves to hold the posture. Rather than the singular flexing action in a particular muscle from lifting a weight, which isolates and strengthens that muscle, yoga poses encourage a coordinated effort among all body parts, muscle, joint, and bone, legs, torso, and arms, to target a particular area. Rather than twelve repetitions that target a particular muscle and bone (the recommended form of weightlifting for people on the Longevity Diet), yoga uses your own body weight by holding the poses for longer periods of time, which stimulates the bone[13] while increasing flexibility in the muscles.

The standing poses provide a full range of movement for the legs and hips, and thus will help to maintain both the stability and flexibility required for a healthy back, strong hips, and limber knees.

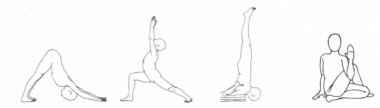

Twists encourage circulation to the intervertebral disks, help to relieve backaches, and will improve elimination. Yoga also releases the muscular tension so often faulted for headaches, indigestion, and sleep difficulties.

Over time you may be introduced to inversions, the infamous headstand and shoulder stand poses. These postures become weight-bearing exercises for the upper body and, in particular, the spine. Because the vertebral column is very susceptible to fractures, and is difficult to isolate in exercise, these postures may be able to stimulate bone density in the spine itself. There are, however, many contraindications to both the headstand and shoulder stand, so it is imperative that you seek out a qualified instructor and begin gradually before attempting to go upside down!

April's Story

I went to yoga for relief from acute anxiety and depression. At the yoga studio I found compassionate, loving, beautiful teachers who taught me how to live in my body. I am not naturally flexible at all, but they taught me to move through the flows and make modifications, and I love being present with myself, my body, and other practitioners.

I began to develop muscle. I started to think of myself as strong. I started to be strong.

I have meditated for more than five years, but always as a medication for what was once a terrifying anxiety disorder. I knew that yoga was tied to meditation, but while my body got stronger and more beautiful and my emotions began to regulate themselves in a more happy-making way, I still didn't connect to the deep inner stillness that is the real point of yoga.

Then I started to work with an Iyengar-trained teacher, Jonathan. He didn't teach dance-y flow-y flows. He taught the poses, broken down into tiny little pieces, and he taught poses that would help us work up to the poses we were trying to learn. He used a lot of props: blocks, blankets, a stretching strap, all to get us close to the correct pose in spite of whatever physical limitations we might have.

A knee injury that I'd had ceased to hurt. My persistent tailbone injury stopped giving me pain. And I started to have these short glimpses of the stillness of the mind.

Iyengar is an exacting style of yoga, and Jonathan is an exacting teacher. But in his classes, I do not see my physical limitations as limitations: I see them as challenges and opportunities. I no longer feel like I have failed because I can't do a pose the way my beautiful flexible yoga teachers can. I feel successful when I work hard, when I take direction well, and when I show up every day. I am gradually starting to love my body again. I know that when I am in class, no longer comparing myself to the other girls with beautiful down dogs, I feel at home in my body and happy to be there. I look at my body as a vehicle by which I travel to those moments when the mind is still. When I am for just one breath present with the essential quiet of the universe.

This love for my body is gradually transitioning into my CR. For a couple of years now I've been practicing healthy eating/obesity avoidance, but I want to do CR because I want to stay young and healthy as long as I can, and eventually catch that bus to radical life extension. Yoga puts me in a space beyond time and space, beyond the separateness of my life as distinct from all life. But it also puts me in a space of deep respect for this living container of my soul, and out of that respect, I find myself going back on hardcore CR.

Not All Yoga Is Created Equal

Today there are as many schools of yoga as there are types of running shoes. Buyer beware: You will find power yoga, yogaerobics, hot yoga—anything that will sell the image of a lean muscle machine. Our purpose here is to build bone strength, improve flexibility, and reduce stress. Trendy styles of nontraditional yoga lack cohesive standards, so your chance of finding a teacher who understands good alignment is hit or miss.

In addition, these popular classes tend to be large and are conducted in heated rooms; sometimes the instructors even teach through headsets. We suggest you avoid yoga teachers or venues that do integrate conscious relaxation. Also, Integral yoga, Sivananda yoga, and the Viniyoga systems place more emphasis on meditation and relaxation so, while they may calm your mind, they will not benefit your bones.

The Iyengar and Anusara systems of yoga have certified teachers trained in good alignment. In particular, instructors teaching under the Iyengar trademark are skilled in both remedial applications of yoga (injuries from other exercise programs) and in overall good form. Even when pursuing these systems, be sure you work with a certified instructor in a supportive space.

Stress—The Silent but Insidious Mole

With so many well-documented ill effects of stress, we are continually amazed at how few people actively pursue relaxation techniques. While exercise is currently a marketer's dream, with the proliferation of fitness studios, gyms, equipment, videos, clothes, and trainers, relaxation is relegated to an afternoon by the pool or a massage. And while increased interest in exercise is a welcome counterpoint to the dire statistics underlining the rise in sedentary lifestyles, including diabetes, hypertension, and obesity, it omits the powerful mind-over-body effect for which conscious relaxation is well known.

Everyone would agree that less stress leads to better health; and that sleep, eating, and mood disorders are often associated with anxiety. Studies show that chronic stress decreases the body's ability to heal, from minor cuts to major surgery. Chronic psychological stress can lead to an accelerated shortening of telomeres (cellular aging; see page 82), as recently reported in a PNAS (Proceedings of the National Academy of Sciences) article.[14] Stress quadruples the risk of asthma attacks in children,[15] and is seen as a cause of some miscarriages. The National Institute of Mental Health distributes a handbook titled *Stress and the Developing Brain,* alerting parents to the dangers of a stressful household to children. Researchers at the Boston School of Medicine contend that acute and chronic stress induces a chronic inflammatory process that culminates in atherosclerosis. These findings may account for up to 40 percent of diagnosed cases that cite no other attributable causes. The list is quite extensive and covers everything from irritable bowel syndrome to exacerbating the painful effects of rheumatoid arthritis and multiple sclerosis.

In addition to supporting the physical healing process, relaxation techniques help reinforce a person's resolve to stick with a healthy lifestyle makeover and to cope with life's changes.

Some stresses are beneficial and others harmful. How can stress be beneficial? Mikhail Baryshnikov once said that he was nervous before each dance performance. Perhaps this is what gave him the edge that made his leaps so breathtaking. Similarly, the intoxication before a romantic evening or the anticipation before a job interview produces the aroused, or heightened, state of consciousness we associate with performance anxiety, and this in turn sharpens our senses. Our adrenaline flows. We become more alert. We are stressed by looking forward to something we want to accomplish, and that very stress can be the boost that helps us achieve it.

Purely physical stress can also be beneficial: In physics, stress is the internal resistance of a body to an applied force or system of forces. As in resistance-training practices and in aerobic exercise, this productive stress triggers the adaptive mechanisms in the body to strengthen internal structures—bones and such systems as the cardiac and respiratory.

But we most commonly associate stress with this dictionary definition: "A mentally or emotionally disruptive or upsetting condition occurring in response to adverse external influences capable of affecting physical health, usually characterized by increased heart rate, raised blood pressure, muscular tension, irritability, and depression." Now, that sure doesn't sound beneficial, does it?

Take care that your attempts to relax do not actually produce additional stress. Some people say that they find prolonged exercise relaxes them, that it solicits a natural high, like "entering the zone." This is different from *choosing to practice* a centering method or relaxation technique that helps you to cope with any increase in pressure, be it from external circumstances or internal issues. To go for a run when you are stressed out may indeed help calm you, but it may wear your resources thin if your anxiety level has persisted for a period of time; you may be more prone to injury and you may lower immunity against illness. How? Stress hormones, along with other deleterious consequences, have a strong anti-inflammatory effect on tissues, muscles, and joints. Hence, you might actually feel like you can do more and that the exercise is enabling you to tune out your feelings, but you are acting *under the influence* of a strong chemical effect, that of excessive adrenaline. If the adrenal glands continue to pump adrenaline into the body, over time they become exhausted, and the neurotransmitters that deliver messages of well-being and restore internal equilibrium become muted. Your immune system then shuts down, and you become vulnerable to physical accidents, even to infection.

Thoughts are food to the mind; and they can nourish or poison you. Every state of mind affects the body, even if you are not conscious of their doing so. If your body pipes up with stress-related symptoms, you need to listen and to find a safe means of releasing your stress. While adequate family and community support or psychological maturity is helpful, for a long and healthy life we encourage you to seek out and practice some relaxation technique, be it meditation, keeping a journal, visualization, or biofeedback. True relaxation techniques enable the mind to let go of obsessive thought patterns and replace them with a composed perspective. In our opinion, the most advantageous thing that you take from this chapter is this understanding of conscious relaxation.

In a pinch, you can quickly realign your runaway reactions before acting impulsively. Try the following:

Close your eyes. Take in a gentle but deep breath, imagine the air nourishing every cell in your body with tranquility, composure. As you exhale, open your mouth slightly and let a satisfying sigh escape your lips. Or you might prefer to relax all the muscles in your face as you exhale, especially the jaw, like chocolate melting in the sunlight.

The Relaxation Response

The relaxation response, a state of deep physiological relaxation, is characterized by a reduction in heart rate, blood pressure, respiratory rate, and muscular tension; many of the effects are similar to those of calorie restriction.

Many methods may induce this effect. Some of us are more visually inclined, so guided imagery may be effective. Some are more kinesthetic, or physically oriented. Progressive relaxation emphasizes the gradual release of all voluntary muscular tension until you experience a deep state of inner peace. Various meditative schools use awareness of the breath as a focal point to shift into an **alpha,** or a heightened, state of consciousness. Pain-management programs often begin with exercises, which first bring awareness to the movement of the breath, and then to deepening the exhalation. Prayer is effective for many, as is the repetition of a simple yet meaningful phrase, which helps train you to shift your mind from scattered thinking to purposeful, controlled, and quiet thought.

As important as what you choose is *how often* you do it. A few minutes every day will be far more effective than a class you take once a week. So begin with something simple, something that you can practice preferably at home. There are many good tapes available, or, if you do find a class, practice! The cumulative effect and skills you reap from this work will help support your commitment to the Longevity Diet lifestyle.

The Yogic Path to Conscious Relaxation

The following yoga postures are especially effective in inviting relaxation. Some yoga poses focus more on stretching and range of motion. These poses passively expand the chest, release tension in the upper body, and free the diaphragm from its habituated heaviness. By passively inflating the chest and releasing muscular tension, you increase the circulation in the upper body while quieting the breath and releasing pressure across the diaphragm and abdominal organs. In restorative work like this, the yoga is doing you, rather than you having to apply yourself to the exercise.

If you have tried meditation, and your mind did everything but relax, this might be a better solution for you. Whereas the fight/flight reaction is almost instantaneous, the relaxation response physiologically takes a little longer to kick in. So you should stay in each pose for seven to ten minutes, especially if you find that your mind runs amok for the first few minutes! It is the natural tendency of the mind to be busy; that is its comfort zone. We either are switched on, thinking, or off, dreaming or sleeping. Mindfulness and conscious relaxation require an alert presence that is wakeful and yet receptive. With time, this state of mind—and it is a real condition of the mind—can become as much a part of your daily experience as analytic, problem-solving, or creative thought. It is frequently referred to as the witness state. But as with building any new behavior, it only works through reinforcement, by practicing.

These three poses can be done anytime of day or night, but preferably not right after eating. They can be practiced in any order, but you will find that each sequence will have a different effect on you. At the end of the day, begin with the Legs up the Wall Pose, and end with the chest lifted and the full body extended in the Supported Corpse Pose. If you choose to anchor your day with conscious relaxation, then practice in the morning and remember to stay serene. Begin with the Supported Corpse Pose. This will gently open the intercostal muscles on the sides of your rib cage to aid you in deep breathing.

Follow the instructions below, but feel free to modify each pose to make it comfortable. Stay warm! As you begin to relax, your body temperature will lower, so have a light-weight blanket at hand. We find it helpful to work with a timer, otherwise you might be tempted to keep watching the clock!

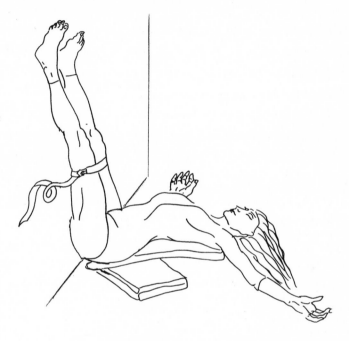

Legs up the Wall Pose: Viparita Karani

Lie face up on the floor or carpet and support your calves on a chair. With your hands, gently lengthen the buttocks away from your lower back to release any tension in the lumbar spine. The weight of the legs should release down into the hip sockets. Place a folded blanket, towel, or pillow beneath your neck and head. Your forehead should be lifted slightly higher then your chin. Relax your arms out to your side, far enough from your body to allow them to roll open. The weight of the arms should encourage the shoulders to release toward the floor. Feel free to cover your eyes with a cloth or an eye bag. Remain here for seven to ten minutes.

Legs up the Wall Pose is helpful to relieve tired or aching legs and feet and to prevent varicose veins; to alleviate mild lower back-aches; to recover from fatigue or jet lag; to prevent migraine and stress related headaches; and to calm the mind.

Variations: In the classic pose, the legs are up the wall and the pelvis is supported by a folded firm blanket or bolster. Elevating the pelvis with a blanket helps to lengthen the abdominal area away from the chest to open the chest and release the diaphragm. When placing the pelvis on the blanket, allow the buttocks to release slightly off the blanket toward the wall, as seen in the picture. If you are stiffer in the hamstrings, shift your body a foot away from the wall so that your legs are on a milder angle and use a smaller blanket fold. This will reduce the hamstring stretch otherwise required of this pose.

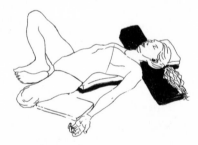

Sweet Space Pose: Supported Sukhasana

Sukha means "happy space" or "sweet space" in Sanskrit. This pose is a favorite and can be practiced anytime, even in bed, as long as you have enough support beneath the spine. The blankets need to be firm enough to lift the chest up evenly and support both sides of the torso and narrow enough to allow your arms to release off of the support. The bolsters on the back of a couch work sometimes, although they are frequently too wide. Two firm blankets folded lengthwise and about six inches wide should work. The legs can be straight, crossed at the shinbones, or bent with the feet touching, depending on your flexibility.

Begin by sitting a few inches away from the blanket support. Cross your legs evenly in the center of the shins, or place the soles of the feet together, as in the picture. Lie onto the blanket-bolster support, leaving a few inches between the support and your buttocks. To release the lower back, lengthen the flesh of the buttocks away from the back of the waist by hooking your thumbs onto the buttocks and sliding the flesh toward your heels. If you feel any stretch in the groins on the inside of the legs, place a towel beneath your thighs, so that your legs can relax.

The blanket/bolster supports and lifts the chest up off the abdominal area. As you open the chest, you will release the diaphragm and passively stretch your auxiliary respiratory muscles, the intercostals. This posture relaxes the digestive tract; relieves constipation, menstrual cramps, and lower backaches; and helps allay anxiety attacks. It is a wonderful tonic at the end of the day!

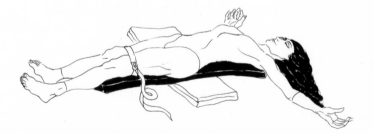

Supported Bridge Pose: Setu Bandha

Place your folded blankets lengthwise on the floor. Lie down on the blankets, with your head beyond the edge of the blankets on the floor, but your shoulders on the blankets. Bend your knees and gently push with your feet until you slide your shoulders off the blanket onto the floor. This sliding action should pull the trapezius muscles away from your shoulders and help to roll the shoulders down toward the floor, so avoid wiggling back onto the floor. Slowly straighten the legs. Release the arms at your sides, far enough from the body so that they naturally release and roll out to the sides. If you feel any discomfort in your lower back, raise the height underneath your feet with a few books or blankets. You may also prefer to use a pillow beneath your head, or a neck roll to support your cervical (neck) curve. Finessing your position in these postures is similar to selecting the right bed, take the time to make it comfortable. Remain here for seven to ten minutes.

This pose is especially good for helping you sleep at night. It calms the brain and helps to alleviate stress, mild depression, lower and upper backaches, headaches, and fatigue.

How Do I Begin My Longevity Exercise Regimen?

Whether you work out with a trainer, go to a gym to use the equipment, or exercise on your own, practice your aerobic and resistance-training programs on alternate days. This will allow your muscles, tendons, ligaments, and joints to recover from any potential excessive use. And remember, aerobic activities, weight-bearing or resistance training, and stress reduction are *all* important elements of a healthy lifestyle. (Remember that the serious and mature practitioner of calorie restriction may have adequate cardiovascular benefits through diet alone.) Do not rely on a single activity; coordinate your schedule to toggle among several.

Here is a sample weekly schedule to help you visualize how these programs can work together:

Sunday: Aerobic activity: walk, hike, skate, run, swim twenty to thirty minutes

Monday: Resistance workout or Iyengar yoga class (or any form
that holds standing poses and inversions)

Tuesday, a.m.: Twenty to thirty minutes of aerobics; p.m.: thirty
minutes of stretching

Wednesday: Resistance workout or Iyengar yoga class

Thursday: Aerobics: a fun, social activity such as skating or bik-
ing, to counteract any midweek slump

Friday, AM: Twenty to thirty minutes of aerobics; thirty minutes
of stretching or resistance work

Saturday: Resistance workout or Iyengar yoga class, or alternate your activities with yet another kind of aerobic activity
or stretching class.

Your present or projected schedule may look quite different,
depending on your preferred routines and available time. If you
already practice yoga, add an aerobic activity (unless your style of
yoga is aerobic). Perhaps, especially if you run, the kinds of warm-
up stretches you already do may not be enough to strengthen all
your bones nor will they help with your tight hamstrings and
upper back; seek out a stretch or yoga class. Whatever you do, be
sure to choose activities that you enjoy, in a setting you like. If
formally structured exercise is difficult to fit into your lifestyle,
remember that active sports, dancing, and even just twenty minutes spent walking up and down the stairs at home or an office
building (find a colleague willing to go "buddies" with you during
a break) are all exercise.

As with your food choices, if you enjoy your physical activities,
you will be more likely to stick with your goals. If you exercise
solely because it is good for you, and not because you like to, your
chances of maintaining a well-balanced program over the long
haul are slim. Perhaps you multitask by reading the newspaper
while using a stationary bicycle or by watching the evening news

while stretching. That's fine. But don't use such tactics to block from your consciousness what you are actually doing with your body. If you really see and appreciate the trees, the sky, and the people around you while you work out, or use your exercise period to tune in to the world inside yourself, with its sensations of breath, warmth, the release of a tight muscle, or the stimulation of a spine unfolding and lengthening, then your exercise regimen will feel gratifying in and of itself and will become an integral part of your life.

Optimal Living from a Few Veteran Practitioners of the Longevity Diet

PETER:

In addition to being an advocate of CR, Peter Voss exemplifies the integration of thought and action that Dr. Walford referred to in his preface to *Maximum Life Span*: "I believe that the effects of life-span extension will be outstandingly positive for mankind as both social and individual animals, will help solve many of our dilemmas, and revolutionize human potential." A longevity diet is but one facet of Peter's vision to enhance what it means to be alive.

Contrary to popular opinion, I see the impending dramatic improvement in longevity as a tremendous boon for mankind. Not only for the obvious selfish benefit of living a vastly extended vital life, but more generally for the advantage of having more wise people active in society. Today, just as we learn how to live life—you know, after three careers and two marriages . . . well, seriously—having learned to be in touch with our emotions; how to effectively communicate with others; how to make and keep money; having raised children; having had the time and interest to study some psychology, philosophy, and science; having developed an appreciation for art, and so on—we find ourselves out of circulation. As our active years are extended, I expect that many more dynamic, wise, and able people will experience and demonstrate Optimal Living—and will thereby positively contribute to society. My passion is for exploring what I call Optimal Living: maximizing both the quantity and quality of life. Optimal Living is not one single, "perfect" version of life. *Optimal* means "best or most favorable under a given set of circumstances." The circumstances and contexts of our lives are also in a continual state of flux. Specific values optimal to one person at a given time may be detrimental in a different context.

Hence, there are many ways to coordinate the factors in CR. CR is a lifestyle change, it is not a diet, and will therefore be unique to each individual. It can be a positive experience— I would focus on finding new and delicious foods and food preparations rather than on what I "shouldn't eat," and I would not beat myself up if I thought I had failed. I made a point of discovering ready-to-eat and easy-to-prepare healthy low-cal foods that I really enjoy—often this simply meant improving the meal by changing the type of dressing used (delicious fat-free versus conventional mayonnaise) or the quantity of some ingredients (half the rice).

As I see it, the basics are simple: Subject to certain limits, the fewer calories you consume, the better your health and longevity, and the benefits are proportional. The primary payoff is avoiding, or vastly delaying, the major killer diseases: heart, stroke, diabetes, cancer; but other benefits include a stronger immune system, increased fitness, and a greater appreciation of food.

In the context of my philosophy of Optimal Living, this also implies that I must enjoy my CR lifestyle—in addition to striving for vastly increased longevity and vitality. Good nutrition and exercise are complemented with strategies for improving mental and financial well-being and for reducing risk of accidental death—plus the ultimate safety net (of unknown fabric): cryonics.

Let's work towards overcoming life's current limitations. Let's have the option of enjoying a fuller, healthier, and much longer life. Who knows what new heights we may reach. . . .

DEAN:

In the formative years of the virtual CR Society, Lisa and Roy Walford regularly observed the CR list while refraining from posting, to avoid any semblance of influencing the generally friendly but sometimes heated milieu of these extremely bright people with strong opinions.

Inspired by the imaginative approaches many practitioners adopted for themselves, they were particularly drawn to the systematic way that Dean applied himself to the Longevity Diet. Dean's is a well-known voice on the CR Society's mailing list, answering sophisticated questions as well as offering simple suggestions to the newcomers who frequent the community.

> This diet has created a life for me here and now that I truly love and find incredibly fulfilling. Any health/longevity benefits that may accompany my practice of CR I consider to be "gravy."

Let me try to explain. As you may be aware, CR results in a number of physical and psychological changes in its practitioners. The usual focus in CR is on how the physical changes impact health/longevity. The psychological changes are typically either ignored or viewed as unfortunate side effects.

What are these psychological changes? I can only speak from personal experience, but I've been told by other people on CR that they've experienced some of these as well. Specifically, I've noticed changes in my brain's "reward centers"—I definitely receive more internally generated positive feedback from little things than I ever did prior to CR. For me, such appreciation of little things started with food.

For example, I eat and have been eating an identical, relatively simple meal three times a day for well over a year. Prior to CR, I could never have imagined such behavior. More interesting, I truly get pleasure from each and every one of these meals. In fact, I'm certain I enjoy my food more today than I ever did prior to CR, despite its monotony.

With some training, finding pleasure in simple things extends into other aspects of life. I would never have anticipated this from CR. It is as if the so-called deprivation in one area of my life (food) has fostered a sense of gratitude and appreciation in all areas, which may need to be experienced to be appreciated, but is a truly wonderful state. Suffice it to say that I hop out of bed each morning anxious to experience what the day has in store, despite the fact that quite often, today is very much like every other day.

CR is not like the Atkins diet or the South Beach diet or the Weight Watchers point system, where there's a very prescribed set of things you can and can't eat. You have to decide how many calories you need, how far you want to drop, what the easiest way to practice is. So your intention is important. Successful veteran CR folk tend to be in it for the adventure. We might think, "If I feed my body the right things, it will work better" as opposed to, "I want to look better." The science of it and the tweaking and tuning of it appeals to a different demographic.

In the beginning, CR did interfere with my enjoyment of life. Food clouded my thoughts for at least a year. Food obsession, long hours spent in food preparation, and thoughts about how to best avoid/delay my own mortality distracted me from things that are (or should have been) really important to me, like my family and helping others. I am the sole practitioner of CR in my family (wife and two young children). I have worked very hard to optimize my practice of CR so as to reap the benefits without compromising my relationship with my family. Mostly this has meant streamlining my food preparation so as not to interfere with my family time.

You might ask: Doesn't the hardship associated with my extreme form of CR detract from my quality of life? Let me try to explain. I've experienced a calming of the emotions and my appreciation of the little things in life started with the diet. Put together with the extraordinary health benefits, CR is well worth it.

I'm happy to report that I remain committed to my vegan version of CR and it has served me very well in the five years since the first edition of *The Longevity Diet* was published. I've moderated my diet just a bit for the "long haul" and have gained back about 8 pounds from my low around 120 (I'm 5'9"). My CR is on auto-pilot now and I'm really finding it a great way to live.

In the past couple years I've experienced several life changing events. Two years ago I sold the startup I'd been building for the previous ten years to a really large and established firm. They had very high-powered attorneys negotiating the deal. It could have been a very stressful experience—an emotional person might have cracked under the pressure or blown the deal by getting upset at their initial "low ball" offer. But the equanimity CR provides allowed me to maintain an even keel during those tumultuous few months. In the end we closed the deal under very favorable terms. I'm convinced the financial security I now enjoy is in large part a result of the "calm abiding" attitude that CR has given me. At 44, I've now started over in an entirely new field (brain science) at a large corporate research lab, and loving it. I'm no longer working for the money—I simply enjoy the intellectual challenges and the camaraderie my new career has to offer.

The second major event was a painful one—the death of my dad. He died last year from a heart attack at age 70 while shoveling snow for my sister—giving to others right up to the end. As you might imagine, it was a very difficult time for me, my family, and especially my mom. But CR's psychological benefits helped me keep a healthy perspective and allowed me to support my family during that very painful time.

In short, CR remains an integral part of my life. I'm convinced it has been instrumental in the success I've been blessed with and has helped me to weather the storms that are an inevitable part of every person's life.

FRANCESCA:

A much-publicized *Washington Post* article did more to put CR on the map than former research reviews in the *Wall Street Jour-*

nal and even the *New York Times*. Why? The story featured two women, their trials and tribulations in life, and finally CR. Francesca was one of these women. Francesca has been an active member of the CR Society.

I'm Francesca Skelton, sixty-four years old, and I started CR-ing in the spring of 2000.

For the vast majority of my life, I was very thin—one of those lucky people who could eat just about anything I wanted, and as much as I wanted, without gaining weight. And I took great advantage of that, often consuming vast amounts of food with no visible consequences!

That all changed in 1999, when my oldest brother died of cancer just six weeks after diagnosis. This was the latest in a string of losses of close relatives due to ill health. I was devastated and stopped eating in my usual hearty manner, and in fact, ate very little for several months as I grieved my brother's death and lost weight—weight which I could scarcely afford to lose. Thankfully, after a few months, I recovered from the grieving process, but my metabolism had completely changed. I started gaining weight for the first time in my life. I discovered I could no longer "pack it away" without gaining. When my 5'4" small-boned frame reached 138, or about twenty-two pounds over my usual lifetime adult weight, I was jolted into the realization that something had to be done. I now weighed more than I ever had in my life.

I turned to CR. Four years later, my weight is 110 to 112 (depending on whether I am soaking wet or not), but even more importantly, I am rarely ever sick. Previously, in a year, I would suffer two colds, and one or two bouts of miserable stomach viruses. These are now all history! My immune system is functioning at a level as never before. I constantly marvel at my resistance to illness.

But there's more. As a bonus, my skin looks great and my hair is full, healthy, and bouncy—this at an age when many woman are starting to experience thinning hair. Certainly CR is worth any small sacrifice for the beauty benefits alone!

Fortunately, I find it easy to stay on CR. If I stray a bit, I just get right back on the program. My "tips" and best catalysts for success are (1) online support; (2) reminding myself of my present good health and how awful it used to feel to be sick; and (3) staying on a moderate program—one that is easy to stick to over the long haul.

LOUISE:

Louise is a marathon runner, yoga practitioner, and Peter Voss's life partner. While the two of them have been regular participants at CR Society International conferences, Louise did not readily adapt to the program. As an athlete, her concerns were different from those of the standard American doubter.

Beginning the Longevity Diet was a long process, and I started with a very modified approach. I decreased my calories very gradually. I was convinced from the beginning that I could not be on CR if I wanted to continue running. The biggest change for me was to realize that just because I run does not mean that I have to eat carbohydrates. And what I mean is potatoes, rice, bread, pasta. When I cut down on these foods, I did not see any decrease in my athletic ability. I did not have to eat a pasta meal before my 14-mile run; a salad was just fine, with a little seared chicken or salmon. That was the biggest change over the years; I have almost totally eliminated the white stuff. It is very rare for me to eat bread or pastries. It is mostly fruit and veggies now.

I weigh myself every day. I am aware, but I am not upset if I gain a few pounds. I fast on Mondays, not so much for the calories, as to develop an appreciation for all the people who grow and transport my food and to develop an inner strength, the mental toughness that I could cope without food in the event of a disaster. But I'm not rigid about it. Of course, the less you weigh, the less calories you need. And as we get older, our metabolism slows down, and I see that I don't have the appetite to eat the huge meals that I ate years ago!

I eat two meals a day. I begin my days with coffee and fruit, all kinds of fruit, berries, melons, oranges, papaya, grapes. Sometimes I'll eat a peanut butter performance power bar. Then for lunch a big dish of steamed veggies, red pepper, broccoli, carrots, squash, sweet potatoes, avocados . . . and I love soups. I do not cook, so I find vendors that have good-quality products. I prefer warm foods: I can't stand ice cream, it is too cold, but soups are great. I skip dinner and often take my yoga class at night.

HELGA:

Helga's induction into the Longevity Diet came firsthand, through Dr. Roy Walford. She assisted him in his research with calorie restriction after his exodus from the infamous Biosphere 2 and learned how to cook and coordinate her meals through his example.

I worked for Roy from 1994 until he died, in 2004. He taught me so much! I was not into the science of it, I could not relate to the abstract stuff, and calorie restriction was just a word to me. It is very scientific, the average person does not know what CR means, and I was a little like that. But once I saw Roy chopping the vegetables and cooking, and when I saw the food, I understood. I learn a lot visually, I saw what I could do.

I became more aware of the healthful aspects of the Longevity Diet, calorie restriction, and that it would delay the diseases of aging. Since there is a certain amount of cancer in my family (two of my sisters had breast cancer and my brother has kidney cancer), I saw right away that instead of walking about being terrified of cancer, I could do something about it, I saw it as an instrument of control over my health. From there on I started paying attention and gradually eliminated bad stuff and saw how good I started to feel. I was not actually counting my calories or watching my BMI. That was all too mathematical for me. To make it easier for myself, I started calling myself a vegetarian, as I know what vegetarians eat—they eat a lot of vegetables! I was basically eating the same diet but telling people I was on a plant-based diet instead of CR.

I like to think that if I am out with other people I don't need to be the person who says "I don't eat that," I like to fit in. Being flexible is important.

But when I am around other people, friends, they listen to you politely. We live it, but they don't know what CR means. I have often thought that if it was a different word, it would be good. The word prevents people from grasping what it is; it is too scientific.

The thing about plugging your calories into a program was a difficult idea; most people do not want a laptop in their kitchen. But when you internalize it, you don't need any of those gadgets. Your body is functioning very well, and it lets you know when you are hungry. And once you get going, I don't think you need to count calories. It should not be a thing that impinges on your lifestyle.

How did I feel? I felt clear mentally, my thinking improved, and I had more control over my moods. I was not as emotional as before and not eating any rubbish. I felt more stable, grounded, and able to deal with life. I began some yoga and meditation classes, which made a big impact on me, to be able to think and not react to people emotionally. Life is pretty good right now!

APRIL:

April's contagious enthusiasm permeates her great stories that chronicle the daily highs and lows of social projections, calories, and body image of a young woman on CR. To see her contributions, visit her blog at http://www.mprize.org/blogs/.

When I first started CR, it was a lifeline. I was going through some hard realizations in my personal life, and I knew I had to make a U-turn before I drove my health off a cliff.

For months, CR was an obsession. It was a game, a puzzle, an imaginary friend, an intellectual challenge, and a new religion. My weight loss liberated me to be not just the pretty girl I had always been (if I do say so myself!) but the American female ideal: young, slim, beautiful. Full of life. Tiny enough to be unthreatening.

In the beginning I worked on changing the composition of my diet to increase protein and good fats, replacing junky carbs, and that was a constant struggle. I thought that I could reach lower calorie levels, but I had to put much more effort into the content of those calories to do so with good nutrition. When I first started playing with the lower calorie levels, I was seduced by the high feeling that I got from very low-cal days, and I lost weight too fast. I got scared when I saw that five pounds had come off in only two weeks. The life-extension benefits seem to evaporate in animals that lose weight too fast, and I don't want to be one of those dead rats! So I broke down and bought a scale and started monitoring my weight.

Over time, my CR became more lax. Dinners out with friends, not measuring my wine as carefully. It was as though I could not control my eating while I was out with friends. The cheese plate called to me . . . I had an extra glass of wine. I wasn't physically active at all, but I hadn't been during early CR either, so I didn't think much of it.

In the fall of 2007, a series of events in my personal life occurred that knocked the wind out of my self-esteem. Combined with what I now recognize to be seasonal affective disorder, these events plus my weight gain (while still quite slim, about 115 on what is a medium-to large-boned frame at 5'2") seemed to destroy my positive body image. .It didn't help that I had been through the ringer with the media. I had woken up one morning to find that Slate.com featured an article accusing me, personally, by first and last name, of having an eating disorder. I received death threats on my blog. All for eating kale! Oh, and for being thin. God forbid that an American woman commit the crime of being thin . . . and God forbid she be anything else. Sisters, don't you sometimes think we can't win?

In 2008 the summer came late but it was very warm as soon as it dawned upon us. I decided to walk into the yoga studio I had passed every day for years, the one right up the block from our house.

What happened to me there set me free. I started yoga for relief from acute anxiety and depression and found that I gradually started to love my body again. I look at my body as a vehicle by which I travel to those moments when the mind is still. This love for my body is gradually transitioning into my CR.

CR is not a destination, it is a journey. There is no perfection, but there is perfection in being where you are now, but eyes firmly fixed on the horizon with a flat back, knowing you're going to step back into a position of extreme strength as your next pose.

We are all leaves of an eternal tree, always looking up, seeking to capture the sun's love and feed it to the earth and be fed in turn by her.

Recipes

Fifteen years ago I wrote *The Anti-Aging Plan* with my father, Dr. Roy Walford. At that time the general lore was that low-fat cooking was the healthy-heart way to go. My recipes had to be low or no fat. That certainly tested my ingenuity at the time, and I am pleased that we now embrace and encourage using healthy oils in our recipes!

The recipes that follow are divided into several categories. Many of us live very busy lives and simply do not have time to cook, or even enjoy cooking. The meals in the first section, Ten-Minute Meals on the Run, can be assembled with very little or no preparation. Alternatively, you may be inspired by your commitment to take the high road to health and are ready to try some nutrient-rich recipes. Fun and Fabulous for the Newbie Cook introduces you to cutting, chopping, and combining ingredients to make these one-dish meals. Finally, Mega-Meals for the Top Chef includes three recipes based on roasting and layering ingredients for superb low-calorie versions of some favorite, classic meals.

A few final suggestions: It will help if you replace eat-on-the-run habits with some structure. Decide ahead of time what you will eat for snacks, and keep plenty of fresh fruit and raw vegetables visible on your countertop.

Pick up foods that will satisfy you. You might find that high-energy density foods such as protein fill you up or that the quantity of food in low-energy-density, high-water-volume foods such as vegetable soups and salads satisfy your hunger. The recipes that follow are mainly the latter variety, but chicken or low-fat cuts of beef can easily be incorporated into them. Wherever possible, I have included instructions if meat or fish would make a good addition.

May your food nourish your body so that your body can be a fabulous and fit instrument to nourish your mind, heart, and soul. Start eating!

Ten-Minute Meals on the Run

One-Dish Meals

How you manage your time is an individual thing; and when you eat and what you eat is even more personal. There is no correct way, in fact—no better or best way to do it. The meals in this section are highly versatile; you can pick your favorite vegetables, protein source, sauce, and marinade. The combinations are endless when you get used to preparing your meals this way.

To save time, purchase vegetables precut or use frozen mixed vegetables. Commercial sauces are easy and tasty but they vary in their calorie content, so you should be sure to read the labels. Remember, it takes all of five minutes to broil or bake salmon or chicken to accompany your plant-based meal.

VEGGIES PRIMAVERA

As with mix-and-match clothing, once you have a good base, accessories can transform a simple bowl of veggies into a fantastic meal in one. Here are a few combinations to choose from. Feel free to combine any healthy, premade sauce with your veggies and protein. Get creative!

500 calories approximately per serving, depending on your choices:
150 calories per veggie base serving
125 calories per protein serving
125 calories per sauce serving
100 calories per optionals serving

A. Veggie base: 1 pound packaged raw, cut, mixed vegetables per person—150 calories
B. Select from one of the following:

SERVING AMOUNT	FOOD	OZ/GRAM WEIGHT	CALORIES
3 oz	broiled salmon or other fish	½ cup/85 gm	150 cal
½ cup	roasted turkey leg	3 oz /70 gm	130 cal
½ cup	chicken breast	3 oz /70 gm	160 cal
⅓ cup	chickpeas/ edamame	2.5 oz/80 gm	95 cal
⅓ cup	tofu	3 oz/80 gm	80 cal

C. Select a sauce:

Sauces can change the flavor and texture of any meal, from spicy and exotic to sweet and crunchy. Do try the simplest accompaniment: a good extra-virgin olive oil and high-quality balsamic vinegar with either herbs or a little spicy mango-habanera sauce. Dressed simply, each vegetable flavor and texture stands upright; from the bright crunch of the green beans to the melt-in-your-mouth richness of the potatoes.

PESTO

Serves 3, 130 calories per serving
Fresh is best, but commercial is easiest.

    3 cloves garlic, peeled
    1 bunch fresh basil, or use half basil, half arugula
    1 tablespoon olive oil
    4 tablespoons Parmesan cheese

With the blades running, drop the garlic into a food processor. Add the basil and olive oil. Process for a minute, or until the basil is finely chopped but not pureed. Add half of the Parmesan cheese and a little more liquid as necessary for a moist consistency. Serve with the remaining cheese.

INDIAN TIKKA MASALA SAUCE

Serves 3, 130 calories per serving
    1 tablespoon olive or coconut oil
    2 cloves garlic, minced
    2 teaspoons grated fresh ginger
    1 onion, minced
    1 jalapeño or serrano chile, seeded and minced
    ½ teaspoon ground cumin
    ½ teaspoon ground coriander
    ½ cup plain nonfat or soy yogurt (optional)

In a small saucepan, heat the oil over medium heat and add the garlic, ginger, onion, and chile. Cook until soft, about 4 minutes. Add all the spices and the yogurt (if using). Stir.

MARINARA SAUCE

There are so many good commercial varieties. Purchase one with a little olive oil. Read the label carefully, as some varieties are high-calorie. To spice it up, heat 1 teaspoon of olive oil in a small pan, add 1 minced garlic clove, the marinara sauce, and 2 seeded and chopped fresh tomatoes. Simmer for 15 minutes.

RANCHEROS SAUCE

Use any commercial fresh salsa. Drain the excess liquid; add 1 tablespoon of olive oil and half of a 6-ounce can of medium-size olives.

D. Optionals

Everyone has a different daily calorie goal. Depending on your goal and personal tastes, you might choose to add any of the following ingredients to the basic recipe. Mix and match complementary ingredients. For instance, a basic oil and vinegar dressing would accompany pasta and feta nicely. Or use olives to add texture to a pesto veggie primavera.

½ cup of cooked soba or other whole-grain noodles: 2 ounces—55 calories
¼ cup feta cheese, crumbled: 1 ounce—75 calories
½ cup seasoned croutons: 2 ounces—90 calories
4 walnuts, chopped: 0.5 ounce—90 calories
8 large olives: 36 grams—40 calories
1 tablespoon grated Parmesan cheese: 5 grams—22 calories

MINUTE MARINADES FOR BROILING CHICKEN OR TOFU

Each recipe serves 2, enough for a ½-pound serving

TOMATO-VINO
Serves 2, 100 calories per serving

3 tablespoons tomato paste
1 tablespoon extra-virgin olive oil
¼ cup dry sherry
1 clove garlic, minced
⅛ teaspoon salt
¼ teaspoon freshly ground pepper

TANDOORI GRILL
Serves 2, 40 calories per serving

½ cup plain fat-free Greek yogurt
1 teaspoon grated fresh ginger
2 cloves garlic, minced
1 teaspoon low-sodium soy sauce
1 teaspoon ground turmeric
¼ teaspoon cayenne, or to taste

CAESAR MARINADE
Serves 2, 100 calories per serving

2 tablespoons light mayonnaise
1 tablespoon Dijon mustard
1 clove garlic
¼ teaspoon Tabasco

SZECHUAN SOY
Serves 2, 120 calories per serving

1 tablespoon low-sodium soy sauce
2 tablespoons pure maple syrup or honey
1 teaspoon grated fresh ginger
2 teaspoons canola oil

GADO GADO: INDONESIAN SALAD WITH PEANUT DRESSING

Serves 2, 400 calories per serving without sauce; 100 calories in ⅓ cup of sauce; factor in 60–200 calories if optional protein is added

This dish is fun to assemble and satisfying to eat. Gado gado is a classic Indonesian dish that combines cooked and raw vegetables with a spicy peanut sauce. Take care to serve the sauce conservatively, as that is where most of the calories lie. But hey, it's peanut butter! Good stuff in small doses. Make it extra special by laying out all the veggies like a mandala.

1 (1-pound) package lettuce
4 cups packaged shredded cabbage (¼ head cabbage)
1 cup bean sprouts
1 (2-pound [1 pound per person]) package mixed sliced vegetables (or
    purchase, wash, and cut yourself: carrots, cauliflower, broccoli)
1 cucumber, peeled and cut into 1-inch pieces
1 red bell pepper, seeded and chopped coarsely
3 green onions
½ leftover baked sweet potato, sliced into thick rounds
1 hard-boiled egg
1 hard-boiled egg white
Fresh lime juice (optional)

Sauce:
2 tablespoons chunky peanut or almond butter
¼ onion, minced finely
1 clove garlic, minced
½ teaspoon shoyu (soy sauce)
Juice of 1 lime
¼ cup water, or ½ (14-ounce tub) soft tofu
½ teaspoon red pepper flakes, or to taste

Optional:
¼ (14-ounce) block raw tofu—60 calories
¼ (14-ounce) block fried tofu—220 calories
½ cup chicken breast—110 calories
½ cup small cooked shrimp, or 3 large cooked shrimp—60 calories

This dish is assembled either on a platter or on individual serving plates. Place a bed of cabbage around the perimeter; next, a layer of lettuce inside the cabbage. You now have the choice to continue to make rings of each veggie toward the center of the plate or assemble it freestyle.

Prepare the sauce: Blend all the ingredients in a small blender.

Place the sauce in the center of the dish and sprinkle fresh lime juice (or a teaspoon of olive oil—50 calories) over all the veggies before serving.

Gado Gado
Calories per serving: 500
Percent of calories from:
Protein: 25
Carbohydrate: 53
Total fiber: 27gm
Total cholesterol: 36 mg

Total fat: 12 g
%Saturated: 12
%Monounsaturated: 15
%Polyunsaturated: 62

Nutritional Profile:
percent of RDA per serving:
Vitamin A: 1,030
Vitamin C: 568
Vitamin E: 77
Vitamin B_{12}: 8
Iron: 48
Calcium: 28
Selenium: 47

CHEESELESS, IF YOU PLEASE PIZZA

Serves 1, 550 calories without avocado, 570 with avocado

The flavors in this kitchen-sink pizza are bright; each vegetable distinguishes itself from the others. You can frequently pick these up already roasted in the hot foods portion of your local supermarket. Otherwise, for a quick dish, use steamed veggies. Replace the tomato sauce with refried black beans, add shredded lettuce, and pour salsa over the vegetables and you have a tostada!

1 medium-size whole wheat tortilla
¼ cup tomato sauce, any flavor, without oil or cheese
1 tablespoon tomato paste
Grilled veggies of choice: zucchini, eggplant, shiitake mushrooms, onions
¼ roasted fresh red pepper, or ¼ small jar roasted red pepper, chopped
Sun-dried tomatoes, soaked to rehydrate, then drained and chopped
4 jumbo black olives, halved
¼ onion, minced
½ cup (about 2 ounces) shredded chicken or baked tofu
Fresh basil leaves, if possible
4 squirts olive oil nonstick cooking spray
¼ avocado, cut into pea-size bits, or mashed (optional)

Preheat the oven to 400°F.
Mix the tomato paste with the tomato sauce. Spread on the tortilla.
Spread the veggies—lots of veggies!—plus the protein and olives over the tortilla.
Spread the avocado and basil leaves evenly over the pizza
Spray the top of the pizza lightly with olive oil.
Bake for 15 minutes. Spread with the mashed avocado, if using.

Cheeseless if you please Pizza

Calories per serving: 550
Percent of calories from:
Protein: 23
Carbohydrate: 42
Total fiber: 12 gm
Total cholesterol: 58 mg

Total fat: 23 g
%Saturated: 20
%Monounsaturated: 49
%Polyunsaturated: 45

Nutritional Profile:
percent of RDA per serving:
Vitamin A: 85
Vitamin C: 240
Vitamin E: 61
Vitamin B$_{12}$: 12
Iron: 41
Calcium: 12
Selenium: 92

Fun and Fabulous for the Newbie Cook

MOROCCAN FEAST

Serves 2, 800 calories per serving

With this generous serving, you will fill both your palate and receive over 50 percent of all your basic RDAs. Lamb is a traditional ingredient in North Africa, and you may choose to add a small serving to the soup pot. Optionally, serve with couscous, millet, or brown rice (remember to factor in those calories).

1 ½ tablespoons olive oil
4 cups vegetable or chicken broth
2 cloves garlic, minced
½ medium-size onion, chopped coarsely
2 stalks celery, chopped coarsely
1 medium-size sweet potato, sliced into 2-inch cubes
1 cup butternut or other winter squash, peeled, seeded, and cubed
2 carrots, sliced into bite-size pieces
¼ cup green beans, sliced into bite-size pieces
1 (8-ounce) can crushed tomatoes, or 2 large tomatoes
2 tablespoons grated fresh ginger
1 tablespoon raisins or currants
1 cup densely packed, washed, and chopped fresh or frozen collard
    greens (thaw if frozen)
½ (15-ounce) can chickpeas, drained

Optional:
Lamb: 1 loin chop, lean only—90 calories
Chicken: ½ cup cooked light meat—110 calories
Couscous: ½ cup cooked (less than ¼ cup dried)—90 calories

Heat the olive oil in a skillet. Add the chopped onions and garlic and stir-fry until translucent.

Add the broth, all the remaining vegetables (except the thawed collards and canned chickpeas, if using), and the spices and ginger. Bring to boil, simmer, and cook uncovered for 30 minutes. Add the frozen collard greens, raisins, and the canned chickpeas in the last 5 minutes.

OPTIONAL COUSCOUS OR MILLET:
Serves 2, 90 calories per serving

   1 cup water
   ⅛ teaspoon salt
   ½ cup whole wheat couscous (available at health food stores) or millet

Couscous: Heat the water to a boil in a 1-quart saucepan. Add the salt and couscous. Stir to mix, cover, and remove from the heat. Let the couscous sit for 5 minutes. Remove the cover, and fluff with a fork to serve.
   Millet: Heat the water to a boil in a 1-quart saucepan. Add the salt and millet. Cover, reduce the heat, and simmer for 10 minutes. Remove from the heat, and fluff with a fork to separate the kernels.

OPTIONAL BROWN RICE:
Serves 2, 150 calories per serving

   1 cup water
   ⅛ teaspoon salt
   ¼ cup brown rice (long-grain, medium-grain, or basmati rice)

Heat the water to a boil in a 1-quart saucepan. Add the salt and rice. Cover, reduce the heat, and simmer for 20 minutes. Check the rice after 15 minutes to make sure the pot does not run out of water. Add 2 tablespoons of water and continue cooking if the rice is not fully cooked or the water has been fully absorbed. When the rice is cooked, remove from the heat, fluff, and serve.

Moroccan Feast

Calories per serving: 800
Percent of calories from:
   Protein: 14
   Carbohydrate: 56
   Total fiber: 26 gm
   Total cholesterol: 3 mg

Total fat: 29 g
   %Saturated: 21
   %Monounsaturated: 57
   %Polyunsaturated: 89

Nutritional Profile:
percent of RDA per serving:
   Vitamin A: 873
   Vitamin C: 171
   Vitamin E: 81
   Vitamin B_{12}: 0
   Iron: 75
   Calcium: 51
   Selenium: 56

HUNGARIAN GOULASH

Serves 4, 650 calories per serving

My mother was a full-blooded Hungarian Jew, so I was introduced to the wonders of paprika. Now I might substitute tempeh for the beef in this recipe, but the principles are the same. With a dollop of yogurt or nonfat sour cream, this meal-in-one packs well over 60 percent of all your RDA for everything except calcium. And it freezes well.

    1 tablespoon olive oil
    2 cloves garlic, minced
    1 cup chopped yellow onions
    ½ pound beef round, lean only, cut into bite-size pieces
    3 tablespoons Hungarian paprika
    3 cubes beef bouillon, dissolved in 6 cups hot water, or 6 cups commer-
        cial beef broth
    2 carrots, cut into 1-inch pieces
    1 medium-size to large turnip or parsnip, sliced into large cubes
    1 medium-size potato, sliced into large cubes
    4 mushrooms, sliced thickly
    1 large red bell pepper, seeded and cut into 2-inch cubes
    1 large green bell pepper, seeded and cut into 2-inch cubes
    2 stalks celery, cut into bite-size pieces
    1 (14-ounce) can diced tomatoes
    1 teaspoon dried thyme
    1 teaspoon dried marjoram
    Pinch of salt (optional)

Heat the oil in a large pot or Dutch oven over medium heat. Sauté the onion and garlic until soft, stirring frequently, about 8 minutes.

Add the cubed beef and paprika and sauté over low heat until the beef browns on all sides, about 10 minutes. Add 4 cups of the broth. Bring to a boil, scraping up any brown bits at the bottom of the pot.

Lower the heat to low and simmer for 30 minutes. Add the carrots and turnips and continue to simmer for 10 minutes. Stir in the potato, mushrooms, peppers, and celery. Add the tomatoes and the remaining 2 cups of broth. Add the herbs and salt (if using). Simmer until the meat and vegetables are tender, about 20 minutes longer.

Optional: Transfer 1 cup of soup to a blender and blend until smooth. Add back to the goulash. If you desire, add 1 tablespoon of nonfat yogurt or low-fat sour cream.

Hungarian Goulash
Calories per serving: 666
Percent of calories from:
Protein: 25
Carbohydrate: 46
Total fiber: 21 gm
Total cholesterol: 64 mg

Total fat: 21 g
%Saturated: 20
%Monounsaturated: 41
%Polyunsaturated: 56

Nutritional Profile:
percent of RDA per serving:
Vitamin A: 605
Vitamin C: 404
Vitamin E: 126
Vitamin B$_{12}$: 163
Iron: 106
Calcium: 21
Selenium: 80

JAPANESE HOT POT

Serves 2, 400 calories per serving

A hot pot is usually a big steaming bowl of tasty broth with many vegetables, some fish or meat (or tofu), and noodles. Although this recipe may take you a half hour to make, not only will your kitchen smell terrific but you will savor the fresh tastes of the Orient. Be sure to use the dried shiitakes; they add a rich flavor to this hot pot.

    4 dried shiitake mushrooms
    4 cups water
    1 tablespoon sesame oil
    1 leek, white part only, sliced into ¼-inch rounds
    ¼ medium-size daikon radish, sliced thinly
    4 button mushrooms, sliced thickly
    1 carrot, sliced into ½-inch rounds
    1 medium-size boiling potato, peeled and cubed
    1 stalk broccoli, florets only, cut thickly
    ½ cup snow peas (about 10)
    1 tablespoon grated fresh ginger
    1 cup shredded napa cabbage
    2 cups bok choy, chopped finely
    1 cup firm tofu (prepared with calcium sulfate, such as Nasoya brand), cubed
    1 heaping tablespoon white miso
    Low-sodium shoyu
    ¼ cup sake (optional)
    1 ounce unprepared soba noodles (about ½ cup cooked)

Optional:
10 clams—85 calories per serving
6 medium or 12 small shrimp—30 calories per serving
2 fillets sea bass—120 calories per serving

Rehydrate the dried shiitake mushrooms in 2 cups of water for about 30 minutes, or until soft; dried mushrooms have a more intense flavor than fresh, so don't substitute. Remove the stalks, then cut the caps into ¼-inch slices. Save the soaking water—you'll be using it later for the soup stock.

Heat the sesame oil in a Dutch oven or large pot, then add all of the veggies except for the napa cabbage and bok choy. Stir-fry to coat all the veggies lightly with the sesame oil. Add the ginger and stir well.

Add the shiitake water, sake, and the 2 remaining cups of water to the hot pot and bring to a boil over medium heat. Add the napa cabbage and bok choy.

Simmer over low heat until the vegetables are tender, about 30 minutes.

Add the noodles during the last 10 minutes. Add the tofu, miso, sake, noodles, and shoyu to taste.

Optional variations:
To prepare the clams, sea bass, and/or shrimp, wash well and drop into the hot pot with the noodles. Simmer for at least 10 minutes.

Japanese Hot Pot

Calories per serving: 400
Percent of calories from:
Protein: 22
Carbohydrate: 48
Total fiber: 18 gm
Total cholesterol: 0 mg

Total fat: 13 g
%Saturated: 10
%Monounsaturated: 14
%Polyunsaturated: 94

Nutritional Profile:
percent of RDA per serving:
Vitamin A: 259
Vitamin C: 154
Vitamin E: 46
Vitamin B_{12}: 0
Iron: 66
Calcium: 45
Selenium: 122

DR. WALFORD'S ETERNAL YOUTH CHILI

Serves 10, 470 calories per serving

My father loved his chili! He would serve it with whole-grain toast, beer, and plenty of chopped raw onions. This recipe originally appeared in *Beyond the 120-Year Diet*, but I am sure that he would be pleased to know that I have resurrected it here.

1 cup dried pinto beans, or 2 (15-ounce) cans
5 cups chicken or vegetable broth
2 cups beer
1 teaspoon dried oregano
8 medium-size tomatoes, seeded and chopped, or 1 (16-ounce) can
    stewed tomatoes
6 dried red chile peppers
5 stalks celery, chopped
1 tablespoon canola or olive oil, or nonstick cooking spray
3 large green bell peppers, seeded and chopped
3 medium-size onions, chopped
10 cloves garlic, minced
½ cup fresh parsley, chopped
½ pound extra-lean ground beef, cut into small cubes
1 pound eye of round steak, fat trimmed, cut into small cubes
1 pound lean pork, cut into small cubes
⅓ cup chili powder
¼ cup ground cumin
2 tablespoons coriander seeds
1 (6-ounce) can tomato paste
1 (8-ounce) can tomato sauce
6 to 8 ounces prepared salsa
1 tablespoon yellow cornmeal or masa harina flour
1 (1-ounce) square unsweetened baking chocolate
¼ cup chili salsa with chopped onions (optional)
2 tablespoons chopped fresh cilantro (optional)
Lime wedges (optional)

If you are using dried beans, soak them overnight in water to cover and discard the soak water.

In a large stockpot, bring the broth and beer to a boil. Add the oregano and beans and simmer for 1 hour.

Puree the tomatoes in a food processor, along with the chiles. Add them to the pot along with the celery.

Oil a nonstick skillet and sauté the bell peppers and onions until tender, stir frequently. Add the garlic and parsley and stir well. Remove from the heat and add to the beans.

Oil the skillet again and sear all the meat, stirring constantly, until browned. Add the meat to the stockpot.

Dissolve the chili powder, cumin, and coriander in a small amount of broth to remove the lumps. Add this mixture to the pot, as well as the tomato paste, tomato sauce, and salsa.

Dissolve the cornmeal in enough water to make a paste and add it to the pot. Add the chocolate and simmer for 45 minutes.

Garnish with chili salsa and onions, cilantro, or lime wedges.

Dr. Walford's Eternal Youth Chili

Calories per serving: 470
Percent of calories from:
Protein: 33
Carbohydrate: 36
Total fiber: 13 gm
Total cholesterol: 67 mg

Total fat: 13 g
%Saturated: 30
%Monounsaturated: 23
%Polyunsaturated: 25

Nutritional Profile:
percent of RDA per serving:
Vitamin A: 210
Vitamin C: 441
Vitamin E: 39
Vitamin B_{12}: 84
Iron: 55
Calcium: 12
Selenium: 42

DR. WALFORD'S ALL-IN-ONE VEGETABLE SALAD

Serves 3, 550 calories per serving

Some veteran Longevity Diet practitioners will recognize this classic. I shared many bowls of this salad with my father. The salad bowl would feed us as a main meal for the first day, and then accompany some protein dish for several more days. This salad is better on the second day: The veggies and beans get richer as they marinade; while other vegetables remain crunchy, and flavorful.

Don't be overwhelmed with the number of ingredients; they only require a lot of chopping. Once you get going, it is a meditation.

Feel free to mix and match any seasonal vegetable that you like.

Add the romaine lettuce right before each serving, so that the lettuce leaves remain crisp.

You may use frozen or canned beans to save some time, but fresh is best! Purchasing prechopped veggies will also save time.

⅓ cup dried chickpeas, or ½ cup canned
⅓ cup dried black-eyed peas or other beans, or frozen edamame
⅓ cup uncooked brown rice
¼ cup uncooked wild rice
1 carrot, cut into bite-size pieces
1 broccoli spear, cut into florets and stalk peeled
1 small sweet potato, cut into bite-size pieces
3 medium-size mushrooms, sliced lengthwise
1 large tomato, or 6 cherry tomatoes, seeded and sliced thickly
1 medium-size red bell pepper, chopped finely
1 zucchini or other summer squash (steamed winter squash works well also), chopped
1 small red onion, sliced into thin strips
½ small head purple cabbage, shredded
½ cup chopped fresh parsley or cilantro
4 to 5 leaves romaine lettuce, torn into large pieces
1 hard-boiled egg, peeled and chopped
Optional: 1 avocado—100 calories per serving

Dressing:
2 tablespoons olive oil
½ cup plain nonfat yogurt
½ (6-ounce) can tomato paste
⅓ cup high-quality balsamic vinegar
Herbs as desired (optional)

Soak the chickpeas and black-eyed peas overnight in water to cover. Discard the soak water and, in a large pot, add fresh water to cover. Bring to a boil. Lower the heat, cover, and simmer for 45 minutes. Add the brown and wild rice to the beans and cook for an additional 45 minutes.

Steam the broccoli stalks and carrots for 4 minutes. Add the sweet potato and broccoli florets to the steamer and continue steaming for another 7 to 10 minutes. Drain and cool the vegetables. Place in a large mixing bowl.

Add the remaining raw vegetables to the steamed veggies. Drain the cooled bean mixture and add to the veggies. Add the hard-boiled egg.

Prepare the dressing: Whisk together the olive oil, yogurt, tomato paste, and vinegar, and add to the salad. Add any herbs you desire and mix thoroughly.

Dr. Walford's All-in-One Vegetable Salad

Calories per serving: 550
Percent of calories from:
Protein: 17
Carbohydrates: 60
Total fiber: 16 gm
Total cholesterol: 71 mg

Total fat: 14 g
%Saturated: 12
%Monounsaturated: 28
%Polyunsaturated: 37

Nutritional Profile: percent of RDA per serving:
Vitamin A: 391
Vitamin C: 398
Vitamin E: 63
Vitamin B_{12}: 27
Iron: 38
Calcium: 25
Selenium: 39

LENTIL-MUSHROOM LOAF

Serves 2, 516 calories per serving

This recipe multiplies easily and it freezes well. You can dress it in many colors, with a red roasted pepper sauce, a spicy beet or mustard green sauce, or a standard tomato sauce (recipes follow).
A single serving of this loaf provides half of your daily protein needs. Truly, lentil loaf is a good alternative if you are trying to cut back on your meat consumption.

  2 teaspoons olive oil
  1 ½ cups dried lentils
  ½ cup uncooked brown rice
  3 cloves garlic
  Pinch of salt
  1 onion, sliced into ½-inch rings, plus ½ onion, diced finely
  1 large portobello mushroom, sliced
  3 shiitake mushrooms
  2 carrots, grated
  ½ (6-ounce) can tomato paste
  ¼ cup black walnuts
  1 egg white, lightly beaten
  1 teaspoon dried marjoram
  1 teaspoon dried thyme
  1 teaspoon freshly ground black pepper
  ½ teaspoon cayenne or Tabasco sauce (optional)

Heat 1 teaspoon of the olive oil in small pot with a tight-fitting lid. Add the garlic and cook for 1 minute over low heat. Add 1 ½ cups of water and a pinch of salt and bring to a boil.

Add the lentils and brown rice, lower the heat, and simmer for 25 minutes, or until tender. Let cool, then mash lightly with a potato masher or fork.

Preheat the broiler. Spray a broiling rack with canola oil and position the onion slices on the rack in a single layer. Lightly spray the onions with oil and broil for 4 to 5 minutes, until slightly blackened. Repeat with the portobello mushrooms slices. Do not let them dry out; they should be juicy. Preheat the oven to 350°F.

In a small skillet, heat the remaining teaspoon of olive oil. Add the shiitake mushrooms and cook until tender, about 5 minutes.

Place half of the cooked lentil mixture in a blender, along with the tomato paste and rice. Puree. The mixture will be very thick. Transfer to a large bowl and mix with the onion mixture and the shiitake mushrooms. Add the herbs, black pepper, and cayenne, and mix well.

Lightly oil an 8 ½ by 4 ½ by 2 ½-inch loaf pan and press the lentil loaf into the pan. (This mixture also makes good veggie-burgers. Use an additional egg white and mold the lentil-mushroom mix into four patties, and cook on an oiled baking sheet to desired doneness.)

Bake for 30 minutes and serve with your desired sauce.

Lentil-Mushroom Loaf

Calories per serving: 516
Percent of calories from:
Protein: 19
Carbohydrates: 50
Total fiber: 20 gm
Total cholesterol: 0 mg

Total fat: 17 g
%Saturated: 9
%Monounsaturated: 25
%Polyunsaturated: 100

Nutritional Profile: percent of RDA per serving:
Vitamin A: 367
Vitamin C: 58
Vitamin E: 51
Iron: 61
Calcium: 11
Selenium: 54

ROASTED RED PEPPER SAUCE

Serves 2, 40 calories per serving

1 (12-ounce) bottle or can roasted red peppers
⅓ cup plain kefir or buttermilk, or ¼ cup nondairy milk
Freshly ground black pepper

Place all ingredients in a blender, puree, and serve.

Or roast your own peppers:
2 large red bell peppers, halved and seeded
1 teaspoon olive oil

Place the peppers skin side up on a roasting rack, and press the pepper down as flat as possible. Spray with olive oil.

Roast for 5 minutes, or until the skin shrivels and turns slightly darker.

Remove from the heat and place in a plastic bag to sweat (veggie bags from the grocery store work well for this).

Remove the outer skins by gently rubbing them off.

Proceed with the rest of the recipe as above.

GREENS SAUCE

Serves 2, 80 calories per serving

1 bunch mustard greens (spicy), or spinach or chard (delicate and sweet),
     thick stems removed, chopped finely
1 teaspoon olive or coconut oil
1 clove garlic, minced
1 (1-inch) piece fresh ginger, peeled and grated
½ fresh chile, or more if you prefer it spicy
¼ onion, diced
½ cup kefir, buttermilk, yogurt, or nondairy milk

If using spinach, steam for 7 to 10 minutes. Chard, mustard greens, and kale take 15 minutes to cook. Remove from the heat, drain, and let cool.

Heat the oil in a medium-size skillet over medium heat. Add the garlic, ginger, and chile. Cook, stirring frequently, for several minutes. Add the onion and sauté over medium heat until the onion is soft.

Add the greens and, stirring frequently, cook for 5 minutes, or until the greens are cooked. Stir in the kefir and adjust the seasonings.

This sauce can be served directly from the skillet, or pureed in a blender.

MUSHROOM SAUCE

Serves 2, 100 calories per serving

½ ounce dried shiitake mushrooms
2 medium-size onions, diced finely
1 teaspoon olive oil
3 cups fresh mushrooms, cleaned, stems removed, and diced finely
1 teaspoon dried marjoram
1 teaspoon dried rosemary
1 teaspoon dried thyme
½ cup burgundy wine
Salt

Bring 1 cup of water to a boil and pour over the dried mushrooms. Soak for 30 minutes. Drain the mushrooms, reserve the soaking liquid for the broth. Remove any tough stems and dice finely.

In a saucepan, heat the oil over medium heat. Add the onions, cover, lower the heat, and cook for 10 minutes, stirring frequently. Add the fresh mushrooms and stir over medium heat until the mushrooms turn fragrant, about 3 minutes.

Add the spices, wine, salt to taste, the reserved soaking liquid, and the shiitake mushrooms. Cover and simmer until the mushrooms are tender, about 10 minutes.

If you prefer a thicker sauce, you can sift a little flour into a small portion of the sauce and return the thickened sauce sample back to the pot.

Everything Lean, Green, and in Between, Veggie Dishes Dressed Up

Henry David Thoreau said, "Shall I not have intelligence with the earth? Am I not partly leaves and vegetable mould myself?"

Indeed, fruits and vegetables should form the foundation of your food pyramid and become the building blocks of your new program. Rich in phytonutrients, vitamins, carbohydrates, healthy fats, fiber, flavor, and color, and for the most part low in calories, a plateful of colorful vegetables looks like an artist's palette and will load your frame with vibrant health. The synergistic effects of many of the nutrients in readily available whole foods obviates pharmaceutical companies' attempts to create supplements of equal value. There is just no substitute for the real thing!

Think of a rainbow, where each color contributes its own unique property toward fighting disease, boosting immunity, resisting the effects of aging, and helping to prevent what might otherwise kill you. Following are some very general benefits of various foods, organized by the phytonutrients associated with particular colors.

Green Vegetables

If your veggie is green, odds are that it contains the compound lutein. Lutein is a carotenoid found in the lens of the eyes, and may protect against eye disease. Dark leafy greens contain calcium and protein, and are a rich source of fiber. One cup of cooked kale or spinach or one broccoli spear feeds your body with over 15 percent of heart-healthy omega-3 fatty acids, a lot of vitamin C, and over 50 percent of the brain-booster vitamin folate. Consider including cancer-fighting cruciferous green vegetables such as Brussels sprouts, broccoli, cabbage, bok choy, and watercress to soups or steamed vegetable dishes.

AFRICAN GREENS

Serves 2, 104 calories per serving

1 bunch collard greens (about 1 pound), thick stems removed, shredded
1 medium-size tomato, seeded and chopped
2 green onions, sliced thinly
1 teaspoon almond or peanut butter
Cayenne

Steam the collards for about 10 minutes, or until tender. Do not overcook. Drain.

Place the greens in a skillet over medium heat. Add the tomato and onions. Cook, stirring, for 3 minutes, until the tomato is soft and crushed.

Thin the peanut butter with ¼ cup of water and add to the greens. Stir well.

Heat thoroughly. Season with cayenne to taste.

Serve with rice, fish, or baked fries.

OJ SPINACH

Serves 2, 100 calories per serving

¼ sweet potato, peeled and chopped into ½-inch cubes
1 large bunch spinach (about 1 pound), well washed and cut into thin
    strips
½ red bell pepper, seeded and chopped
1 teaspoon olive oil
1 tablespoon frozen orange juice

Steam the sweet potato for 5 minutes, then add the spinach. Steam
for another 5 minutes, then add the red pepper. Steam for 2 minutes. The
pepper should be crunchy.

Drain and toss with the olive oil and orange juice.

GARLIC GREENS

Serves 2, 100 calories per serving

½ tablespoon olive oil
3 cloves garlic, minced
½ onion, chopped finely
½ teaspoon dried oregano
½ teaspoon dried marjoram
½ teaspoon paprika
1 large bunch beet greens or spinach, or any other greens (about 1
    pound), stems removed, chopped finely
Seasonings suitable to other greens: kale: thyme, basil; mustard greens:
    coriander, turmeric; chard: marjoram, oregano

Heat the oil in a large skillet and sauté the garlic and onion over
medium heat for about 5 minutes

Add all the herbs and paprika, and stir in the greens. Stirring frequently, cook until wilted, depending on the greens used. If you are
preparing kale or collard greens, you will need to add ¼ cup of water,
as these greens take a little longer to cook.

Optional variations:

For spinach, add 1 teaspoon per serving toasted pine nuts or sunflower seeds.

For kale, mix in ⅓ cup of white beans and dried garlic flakes.

For chard, use roasted sesame oil and add 1 teaspoon of roasted
sesame seeds.

ROASTED BROCCOLI WITH GARLIC CHIPS

Serves 3, 75 calories per serving

    1 head broccoli, cut into 2-inch florets, stalks peeled and cut into bite-size
        pieces
    4 cloves garlic, sliced thinly
    ½ teaspoon olive oil
    Freshly ground black pepper
    ¼ teaspoon dried marjoram or oregano

Preheat the oven to 350°F.

In a small bowl, toss the broccoli and garlic with the olive oil. Season the broccoli with pepper and your herb of choice. Spray a baking dish with olive oil and arrange the broccoli mixture in the dish in a single layer.

Roast until the broccoli's edges begin to brown and the stems are tender, about 20 minutes, stirring at the 10-minute mark.

GREEN MACHINE

Serves 2, 160 calories per serving

Years ago, I frequently ate a dish called Bueller's Broth that was considered nutritious and easy to digest. Steam, puree, and you have a wholesome soup that stands alone or can accompany any main course. I supercharged the basic combination with kale and turnip greens to boost vitamin E, calcium, and fiber.

    1 pound green beans, ends trimmed
    2 stalks celery, cut into large pieces
    1 bunch kale (about 1 pound), stalks removed, chopped
    1 cup chopped fresh or frozen turnip greens
    5 zucchini, cut into large pieces
    1 bunch fresh parsley
    ½ lemon or lime, juiced

Steam the beans, celery, and kale for 5 minutes.

Add the zucchini and parsley and steam for another 3 minutes.

Let cool and puree in a blender or food processor, blending in the lemon juice.

Orange/Yellow Vegetables

The warm sunset-colored vegetables such as pumpkins, squash, carrots, cantaloupe, and apricots are rich in beta-carotene, which can help reduce the risks of cancer and heart disease. These carotenoids and the high amounts of vitamin C found in the warm-hued fruits and vegetables boost immunity, may help stave off infections, and reduce inflammation. Citrus fruits, along with orange and yellow fruits such as cantaloupe and papaya, will help to strengthen your tendons and bones.

ORANGE-GLAZED CARROTS

Serves 4, 100 calories per serving

I love carrots steamed with a little drizzle of olive oil, but for guests I will invest a few more minutes for that unusual surprise flavor, in this case, ginger.

- 1 tablespoon coconut oil (substitute olive if you do not have coconut)
- ¾ cup orange juice
- 1 tablespoon fresh ginger, minced
- 8 carrots, peeled and sliced into ¼-inch chunks

Heat the coconut oil over low heat. Add the orange juice and ginger and bring to a boil over medium heat.

Lower the heat and add the carrots. Simmer, uncovered, for 10 minutes, or until the carrots are tender and glazed.

SPAGHETTI SQUASH WITH GARLIC SAUCE

Serves 4, 140 calories per serving

So named for the resemblance of the orange squash strands to spaghetti noodles, spaghetti squash is easy to prepare and very versatile. I have substituted half spaghetti squash for noodles and even prepared an entire pasta primavera with spaghetti squash instead of noodles. Here is a simple spicy olive oil dressing.

    1 spaghetti squash
    1 ½ tablespoons olive oil
    4 cloves garlic
    2 teaspoons red pepper flakes
    ¼ cup pine nuts

Preheat the oven to 350°F.

Slice the squash in half, pierce the skin a few times with a fork, and place face down on an oiled baking sheet. Bake for 30 minutes. The strands should be cooked but still al dente, not mushy.

In a small skillet, heat the olive oil over medium heat. Add the minced garlic and cook, stirring, for 2 minutes. Add the red pepper flakes.

Roast the pine nuts in the same oven while you are baking the squash.

Take a small baking dish (any size, a loaf or casserole dish) and spread out the pine nuts in one layer. Roast for 7 to 10 minutes. Pine nuts will roast quickly, as their fat content heats the nut up quickly.

Remove the squash from the oven and let cool for 5 minutes. While still hot, spoon the spaghetti strands out of the squash shell and mix with the garlic mixture in a serving dish. Sprinkle the pine nuts on top.

SWEET POTATO FRIES

Serves 2, 115 calories per serving

This recipe works with russet potatoes as well. My husband loves them!

Olive or canola oil nonstick cooking spray
2 medium-size sweet potatoes (red-skinned, often called yams) or russet
   potatoes, cut into ¼-inch-thick wedges, peel on
Flavorings of choice: freshly ground black pepper, marjoram, thyme,
   cayenne, nutritional yeast, low-sodium soy sauce, or garlic powder

Preheat the oven the 350°F. Spray a cookie sheet with oil.
Place the wedges on the cookie sheet and spray lightly with oil.
Sprinkle with your desired flavoring(s) and bake for 10 minutes. Turn
the wedges over, spray again lightly with oil, and bake another 5 to 10
minutes, until tender.

BROILED YELLOW CROOKNECK SUMMER SQUASH

Serves 2, 70 calories per serving

This basic formula works for most vegetables. Zucchini is more readily
available, but yellow crookneck squash is so much sweeter!

2 large yellow crookneck squash or zucchini, halved
Olive or canola oil nonstick cooking spray
1 teaspoon olive oil
1 clove garlic, minced
1 tablespoon lemon juice
1 green onion, white part only, minced
½ teaspoon dried marjoram
¼ teaspoon freshly ground black pepper
1 tomato, seeded and cut into wedges

Preheat the broiler.
Spray a baking sheet with the nonstick cooking spray. Place the
squash skin side down on the baking sheet. Lightly spray the squash with
nonstick cooking spray. Broil the squash for 8 to 10 minutes, or until a
fork easily pierces the flesh.
In a large bowl, whisk the olive oil and lemon juice. Add the green
onion, marjoram, and pepper, and mix well. Toss the zucchini and
tomato in the marinade and mix until all pieces are evenly coated.
Place the vegetables on the baking sheet and broil for 7 to 10 minutes,
until the squash is tender. Serve with fish or baked tofu or tofu scramble.

CORN SALSA

Serves 2, 130 calories if veggies only, 160 with shrimp added, 200 with black beans added

1 cup fresh or frozen corn
½ cup celery, chopped finely
½ cup red bell pepper, chopped finely
½ cup red onion, chopped finely
½ cup black beans or small shrimp
1 jalapeño, seeded and minced
Juice of 1 lime

Mix all the ingredients together and let sit for at least an hour to meld the flavors.

PAPAYA RELISH

Serves 2, 80 calories per serving

½ red onion, minced
1 red chile, minced
¼ cup fresh mint leaves, minced
1 medium-size papaya, peeled, seeded, and sliced into bite-size pieces
½ cup red bell pepper, chopped finely
2 tablespoons lime juice

Combine all the ingredients and chill, in the refrigerator, for at least 2 hours.

Purple Vegetables

Blue and purple fruits and vegetables contain phytonutrients called anthocyanin. *Anthos* stems from the Greek word for "flower," and *cyan* derives from the Greek root word *kyanos*, or "blue." Anthocyanin is responsible for the richly concentrated pigment in the skins of berries, grapes, figs, and eggplant. It is a strong antioxidant that helps reduce the risk from heart disease. It may also prevent diabetes and improve cognitive abilities related to the aging brain. In addition, fresh and dried plums and figs are great sources of fiber.

EGGPLANT EAST AND MIDDLE EAST

1 eggplant

Preheat the oven to 400°F.
Pierce the eggplant skin several times with a fork and place in the oven.
Bake for 1 hour. Remove from the oven and let cool. The skin should peel easily and the eggplant is ready for either of the preparations below.

INDIAN STYLE:
Serves 4, 80 calories per serving
Serve this dish with chicken masala or as a spicy sauce to pour over steamed veggies.

1 teaspoon oil
1 teaspoon black mustard seeds
1 clove garlic, minced
1 onion, chopped finely
1 eggplant, prepared as above
4 hot green chiles, or to taste, seeded and minced
2 tomatoes, skinned, seeded, and chopped, or 1 (8-ounce) can peeled
    tomatoes
½ teaspoon turmeric
Salt

Heat the oil in a large skillet over medium heat and add the mustard seeds. When they begin to pop, add the garlic and onion. Cook for 5 minutes, or until the onions begin to soften.
Mash the eggplant with a fork or in a food processor and combine with all the remaining ingredients, season with salt to taste.

MIDDLE EASTERN STYLE: BABA GANOUSH

Serves 4, 80 calories per serving

This classic makes a great dipping sauce with raw vegetables or a good side dish with chicken. Flavor or garnish with mint, parsley, chili powder, pomegranate seeds, paprika, or cumin.

    1 eggplant, prepared as above
    4 tablespoons lemon juice
    1 tablespoon tahini (sesame butter)
    1 clove garlic
    Salt

Puree all the ingredients in a food processor for a smooth texture, or mash the eggplant by hand in a large bowl and then add remaining ingredients, seasoning with salt to taste.

Serve with pita pockets and sliced carrots, radishes, or other raw veggies.

SWEET-AND-SOUR CABBAGE

Serves 4 to 5, 130 calories per serving

This dish can be served hot or cold; the flavors meld overnight.

    1 teaspoon olive oil
    1 onion, sliced thinly into half-moons
    1 small purple cabbage, finely shredded (9 to 10 cups)
    1 tablespoon brown sugar or pure maple syrup
    ½ cup red wine
    ½ cup orange juice
    1 apple, peeled, cored, and chopped finely
    ½ teaspoon ground allspice

Heat the oil in a large, heavy skillet over medium heat. Add the onion and cabbage and fry for 3 to 5 minutes. Add the sugar, wine, and orange juice, cover, and cook for 15 minutes. Add the apple and allspice and continue to cook for another 15 minutes, or until the cabbage is wilted. Check occasionally and add water as needed if the liquid has evaporated.

BORSCHT

Serves 4, 270 calories per serving
This is one of my favorite recipes of all time. I include it under the purple vegetables only because I use purple cabbage, but traditionally it is made with green cabbage. I have also added shiitake mushrooms as an alternative to the traditional beef. A food processor will speed up the preparation time, but consider grating all the veggies good exercise!

½ large head purple cabbage, grated
2 medium-size potatoes, cut into 1-inch cubes, or a dozen little purple potatoes
1 stalk celery
1 bay leaf
2 teaspoons olive oil
1 clove garlic, minced
6 medium shiitake mushrooms, sliced into 1-inch pieces
2 medium-size beets, grated
3 carrots, peeled and grated
Juice of 1 lemon
½ (6-ounce) can tomato paste (about ⅓ cup)
1 cup canned white beans
1 teaspoon freshly ground black pepper
1 teaspoon Hungarian paprika
½ teaspoon fresh dill
Salt
1 cup nonfat yogurt or nonfat sour cream

Heat 6 cups of water in a large pot. Add the cabbage, potatoes, celery, and bay leaf. Bring to a boil, lower the heat, and simmer for 20 minutes.

Heat 1 teaspoon of the olive oil in a skillet and add the garlic. Once the oil is flavored with the garlic, add the shiitake mushrooms. Cover and allow the mushrooms to cook in their own juice, stirring frequently. When the mushrooms are soft, add them to the cabbage.

Heat the remaining teaspoon of olive oil in a large skillet. Sauté the grated beets for about 3 minutes, then add 1 cup of water. Add the grated carrots and bring the water to a boil, lower the heat, and simmer, covered, for about 15 minutes, or until soft. Add the lemon juice and stir well.

Add the cooked vegetables to the cabbage. Add all remaining ingredients and simmer for 10 minutes.

Red Vegetables

Red apples, beets, pomegranates, strawberries, tomatoes, red cherries, cranberries, peppers, and watermelon: Red is vibrant, bold, and rich in flavor. Apples are a great low-calorie high-fiber snack and are versatile in meal planning. They help to lower blood pressure and protect against circulatory problems, while the polyphenol compounds found in the apple peel probably help inhibit the growth of many cancer cells. The lycopene found in tomatoes, watermelon, pink grapefruit, and especially concentrated in tomato sauce and tomato paste helps to protect against lung and prostate cancer.

ROASTED BEETS

Serves 4 to 6, 70 calories per serving

    3 large or 4 medium-size red beets
    Juice of 1 lime or lemon
    1 teaspoon cumin seeds, roasted
    ½ teaspoon ground cardamom
    ¼ teaspoon freshly ground black pepper
    1 tablespoon olive oil

Preheat the oven to 350°F.

Wrap the beets tightly in aluminum foil; you would not want the beet blood to leak! Roast on a baking sheet until tender, about 1 hour. Remove from the foil and let cool, about 15 minutes.

When beets are cool enough to handle, peel them by rubbing off the skins. Discard the roots and stems, and cut into bite-size chunks.

Toast the cumin seeds in a small skillet over medium heat until their aroma fills the air. Remove them from the heat and slightly crush them with a fork. Mix all the remaining ingredients with the cumin seeds and use the mixture to marinate the beets in a bowl.

ROASTED RED PEPPER DIP

Makes 1 ½ cups of dip; serves 6, 120 calories per serving

  1 slice day-old whole-grain bread
  3 red bell peppers, roasted, skinned, seeded, and chopped, or 1 (12-
      ounce) can roasted red peppers
  2 ancho or other mild chiles, or 1 (4-ounce) can
  4 cloves garlic, minced
  ½ cup walnuts, chopped
  2 tablespoons balsamic vinegar
  Juice of ½ lime or lemon
  ½ teaspoon sugar or pure maple syrup, or to taste
  1 tablespoon olive oil

Blend all the ingredients but the oil in a food processor until finely chopped. With the motor running, drizzle in the olive oil until it forms a fine paste.

Serve with celery, romaine lettuce, carrots, or pita bread.

ACE IN APPLES SMOOTHIE

Serves 1, 260 calories per serving

This smoothie served hot makes a rich autumn soup. Served cold, it will fill you up, refresh and nourish you. Whip it with the maple syrup and serve as a dessert.

  1 apple, cored
  ¼ cup cooked winter squash
  ¼ cup canned pumpkin puree
  ½ carrot, cut into chunks
  1 (½-inch length) fresh ginger, grated
  ½ cup nonfat vanilla yogurt
  ½ cup apple or orange juice
  1 teaspoon pure maple syrup (optional)
  Ground cinnamon and/or nutmeg

Blend all the ingredients together until smooth.

Salads

MEDITERRANEAN SALAD

Serves 3, 110 calories per serving
Traditionally, fresh tomatoes add juicy volume to this classic salad, and are a fine substitute. The sun-dried tomatoes add a rich surprise burst of flavor when mixed with the crunch of the peppers.

3 slices sun-dried tomato
1 medium-size red bell pepper, seeded and diced finely
1 medium-size green bell pepper, seeded and diced finely
1 medium-size yellow bell pepper, seeded and diced finely
1 carrot, diced
1 medium-size cucumber, peeled, seeded, and chopped finely
3 cloves garlic, minced
2 green onions, green tops removed, chopped finely
1 small bunch fresh cilantro, chopped
1 teaspoon fresh dill
1 tablespoon chopped fresh mint leaves
1 serrano chile, minced (optional)
1 tablespoon olive oil
Juice of 1 lemon or lime
Freshly ground white pepper

Soak the sun-dried tomato for 10 minutes in water and dice finely.
Combine all the vegetables in a large bowl and add the garlic, green onions, cilantro, and mint. Add the chile, if using, and mix thoroughly.
Drizzle in the olive oil and lemon juice, season to taste with white pepper, and toss well.

TABBOULEH

Serves 3, 115 calories per serving

½ cup raw bulgur wheat
1 bunch green onions, sliced thinly
1 large cucumber, peeled, seeded, and diced
3 tomatoes, seeded and diced
½ teaspoon ground cumin
1 large bunch fresh parsley, minced
1 large bunch fresh mint, minced
Juice of 2 lemons
1 teaspoon olive oil
1 tablespoon finely ground flaxseeds (optional)

Place the raw bulgur in a bowl, cover with cold water, and leave for 30 minutes. Drain the bulgur through a sieve and press lightly to remove the excess liquid.

Mix the green onions with the bulgur and knead lightly with your hands. Add all the remaining ingredients, including the olive oil and lemon juice.

Serve on a bed of lettuce garnished with lemon wedges, tomato, and cucumber.

RAINBOW SLAW

Serves 4, 120 calories per serving, without peanut dressing, 180 with dressing

2 cups shredded green cabbage
2 cups grated carrot
1 cup seeded and finely chopped green bell pepper
1 cup finely chopped celery
½ cup finely sliced cauliflower florets
½ cup finely sliced red onion
½ cup grated beets

Dressing:
2 tablespoons peanut butter
1 teaspoon tamari
1 teaspoon grated fresh ginger
1 teaspoon pure maple syrup
¼ to ½ cup warm water

Mix the salad vegetables together.

Prepare the dressing: Combine the dressing ingredients, using ¼ cup of water, and stir well. If the dressing is too thick, add a little more water.

Toss the vegetables lightly with the dressing.

BEJEWELED SALAD

Serves 5, 150 calories per serving

1 cup cooked brown rice
2 tomatoes, peeled and seeded
1 cup corn niblets, sliced off the cob
½ medium-size cucumber, peeled, seeded
¼ daikon radish, or 8 small red radishes
1 medium-size red bell pepper, seeded and chopped finely
1 medium-size green bell pepper, seeded and chopped finely
½ cup green peas
½ cup chopped celery
½ cup fresh parsley, minced

Dressing:
1 small hot pepper, seeded and minced
2 tablespoons olive oil
1 teaspoon yellow asafetida powder

Combine the rice and all the vegetables in a bowl.
Prepare the dressing: In a separate bowl, mix the hot pepper, olive oil, and asafetida. Toss the rice salad with the dressing.
Dress each plate with a few lettuce leaves, then mound with the rice mixture.

BLACK, RED, AND GREEN SALAD

Serves 2, 150 calories per serving

1 red bell pepper, cut in half and seeded
1 small head romaine lettuce, torn into bite-size pieces
1 small head Belgian endive, cut into bite-size pieces
1 stalk celery, sliced thinly
1 (15-ounce) can chickpeas (garbanzo beans)
½ cup olives
¼ cup toasted walnuts
2 teaspoons non- or low-fat salad dressing of your choice

Preheat the broiler. To roast the red pepper, arrange the pepper halves skin side up on a baking sheet covered with foil. Place the pepper under the broiler for about 5 minutes. Check to ensure that the skin does not burn. When the skin blisters, remove and place in a paper or plastic bag. Seal the bag and let the pepper cool for about 5 minutes. Then, rub the skin off the pepper. Cut the fragrant sweet flesh into pieces the size of a thumbnail.
Combine with all the remaining ingredients and mix well.

MegaMeals for the Top Chef

ROASTED VEGETABLE GRATIN

Serves 4, 450 calories per serving

This dish is a gift from a very dear friend of mine, a fellow yoga instructor who happens to be a top chef. I love talking food with him, and it is out of appreciation for the art of cooking, not out of hunger! People on CR can experiment with fabulous recipes to create novel dishes. This recipe is not as labor intensive as it might appear, short of a lot of cutting and slicing. And although the fat content is higher than some of the other recipes, at 400 calories per serving of gratin, you can afford to add steamed greens or a salad to dilute the calorie-rich gratin by adding green volume to the meal.

2 medium-size Yukon Gold potatoes, cut into ¾-inch chunks
8–10 ounces butternut or banana squash, peeled and cut into ¾-inch chunks
6 ounces portobello mushrooms (2 large), stems removed
1 medium-size eggplant, cut into ¼-inch slices
2 tablespoons fresh basil, chopped finely
2 tablespoons fresh thyme, chopped finely
2 zucchini, sliced into ⅜-inch diagonal strips
2 tablespoons olive oil, or olive oil nonstick cooking spray
1 yellow bell pepper, seeded and diced into ¼-inch pieces
½ medium to large red onion, peeled and cut into ¼-inch dice
4 shiitake mushrooms, stemmed, cut into chunks
8 ounces nonfat ricotta cheese
2 ounces Parmesan cheese (preferably Parmigiano-Reggiano)
1 ½ cups store-bought or homemade tomato sauce
½ (6-ounce) can tomato paste
¼ cup wheat germ

Preheat the oven to 375°F.

Group the potato, squash, eggplant, and Portobello mushroom by vegetable (do not mix together) on a nonstick baking pan and brush or spray with olive oil. Season with a sprinkling of the herbs, and bake for approximately 30 minutes. Let cool. After they have cooled, slice the portobello mushrooms into ¼-inch pieces.

While the potato mixture cools, arrange the zucchini slices on the baking sheet and brush or spray with oil. Season with the herbs and roast for 15 minutes.

Heat 1 teaspoon of olive oil in a medium-size nonstick skillet or spray generously with olive oil spray. Sauté the yellow pepper until half done, about 3 minutes, season with the herbs, transfer to a bowl, and let cool.

Sauté the red onion and shiitake mushrooms in oil until half done, season with the herbs, and let cool.

Mix the ricotta cheese in a bowl with about 1 tablespoon of the Parmesan cheese and the herbs; set aside.

In a separate bowl, mix the tomato paste with the tomato sauce and add the wheat germ.

Assembly: Take a casserole dish and spread approximately 6 ounces of the tomato mixture across the bottom. Layer the potatoes in the bottom of the casserole, then the squash, then half of the cheese mixture.

Take another 6 ounces of tomato mixture and layer it on top of the ricotta. Add a layer of eggplant. Mix the pepper and shiitake mixture together and spread on top of the eggplant.

Add a layer of the remainder of the ricotta mixture, then the portobello mushrooms, then the remainder of the tomato mixture.

Layer the zucchini decoratively on top and sprinkle with the remaining Parmesan cheese. Place a pan under the casserole dish when baking to catch any drips.

Bake, uncovered, for 45 to 60 minutes at 375°F.

Roasted Vegetable Gratin

Calories per serving: 450
Percent of calories from:
Protein: 27
Carbohydrates: 20
Total fiber: 9 gm
Total cholesterol: 30 mg

Total fat: 17 g
%Saturated: 35
%Monounsaturated: 27
%Polyunsaturated: 24

Nutritional Profile:
percent of RDA per serving:
Vitamin A: 145
Vitamin C: 157
Vitamin E: 62
Vitamin B$_{12}$
Iron: 27
Calcium: 36
Selenium: 54
Zinc: 30

SOUTH BY SOUTHWEST LASAGNE

Serves 4, 550 calories per serving

Even lasagne can be low calorie and nutritious, if you choose the right vegetables and add a few super-ingredients, such as tomato paste. This recipe teeters between Southern succotash with kale or collards and the Southwest flavors of fajitas with refried beans and roasted peppers. Each layer is unique and rich.

Besides intuition, practice, and refined taste buds, what makes a top chef? Preparation. While this may seem like many ingredients, if you place everything you will need in the order that you will use it before you begin, the process will go smoothly.

> 2 red bell peppers, cut in half and seeded, or 1 (8-ounce) can
> 1 yellow bell pepper (or green if there are no yellow), cut in half and seeded
> 1 medium-size onion, quartered
> 1 (3-ounce) can mild green chiles
> 3 tablespoons plus 1 teaspoon olive oil
> 10 cloves garlic, minced
> 1 bunch kale, tough stems removed, chopped
> 1 ½ cups commercial tomato sauce
> 8 ounces tomato paste (1 ¼ cans)
> Dash of Tabasco or other hot sauce, or to taste
> 1 fresh tomato, seeded and chopped
> 1 tablespoon dried oregano
> 1 tablespoon dried cumin
> 1 tablespoon dried marjoram
> 1 tablespoon freshly ground black pepper
> 2 long whole wheat lasagne noodles
> 1 (13-ounce) can refried black or pinto beans
> Niblets from 2 ears of corn, or 1 (10-ounce) can
> ½ cup cottage cheese
> ¼ cup wheat germ
> 4 ounces cheddar cheese, grated

Preheat the broiler. Have ready a baking sheet and a 9-inch square baking dish.

Lay the bell peppers skin side up on the baking sheet. Place the onion quarters on the baking sheet. Broil until the skin on the peppers blackens. Remove the peppers and place in a paper or plastic bag to sweat. Set the onions aside.

Turn off the broiler and preheat the oven to 350°F.

Once cooled, remove blackened skin of the peppers by rubbing with your fingers, then chop the peppers coarsely. Mix all the peppers together, including the canned green chiles. Set aside.

Heat 3 tablespoons of the olive oil in a large skillet over low heat. Add almost all the minced garlic to flavor the oil. Add the kale. Sauté, stirring frequently, until all leaves are covered with oil. Add ¼ cup of water, cover, and simmer for 20 minutes, stirring occasionally.

Place 1 teaspoon of the olive oil in a small saucepan over low heat. Add the remaining minced garlic, the tomato sauce, tomato paste, and a little Tabasco. Simmer for 10 minutes. Add the fresh tomato, the cumin, and half the herbs and continue to simmer.

Heat a pot of water over medium heat until it boils. Add the lasagna noodles. Boil for 10 minutes, or until barely tender. Drain, cool, and cut into eight sections.

Heat the beans in a small pan and add the corn and the remaining herbs. Stir to mix. If you prefer a spicy dish, add extra Tabasco.

Assembly: In the 9-inch square baking dish, spread the kale, one layer of noodles (place one square into each of four quadrants), the bean mixture, another layer of noodle squares, the cottage cheese, the wheat germ, and on top, the pepper mixture. Spoon the tomato sauce over everything. Sprinkle the cheddar cheese on top.

Bake for 30 to 40 minutes at 350°F.

South by Southwest Lasagna

Calories per serving: 530
Percent of calories from:
Protein: 21
Carbohydrate: 53
Total fiber: 29 gm
Total cholesterol: 19 mg

Total fat: 16 g
%Saturated: 25
%Monounsaturated: 25
%Polyunsaturated: 35

Nutritional Profile:
percent of RDA per serving:
Vitamin A: 466
Vitamin C: 373
Vitamin E: 103
Vitamin B_{12}: 84
Iron: 52
Calcium: 35
Selenium: 75
Zinc: 34

SPANAKOPITA, SPINACH PIE

Serves 4, 464 calories per serving

This extravagant dish is actually quite simple to make. The fine and flaky pastry that we identify with baklava is called phyllo, or filo, meaning "leaf," or sheet. Although the leaves are delicate, if you follow the instructions included with each box of phyllo, it is quite easy to use. When each sheet is sprayed lightly with olive oil, layered, topped with filling, and baked, the pastry comes out elegant, light, and flaky. You will generally find the sheets in the freezer section of your market. If you are a strict vegetarian, you can omit the eggs from this recipe.

2 medium-size sweet potatoes
1 medium-size butternut squash
Olive oil nonstick cooking spray
2 red chiles, minced
4 cloves garlic, minced
1 large onion, diced finely
2 tablespoons grated fresh ginger
2 large bunches fresh spinach, well washed and chopped, or 2 (10-ounce) packages frozen
1 bunch mustard greens, chopped, or 1 (10-ounce) package other frozen greens
2 teaspoons ground cumin
Pinch of salt
2 egg whites
1 (14-ounce) tub firm tofu, or 1 cup feta cheese
4 tablespoons chopped walnuts
2 tablespoons ground flaxseeds
1 pound phyllo dough (you won't use the whole box; you will need twelve 16-inch square sheets)
12 ounces nonfat cottage cheese, drained as much as possible

Preheat the oven to 350°F. Spray a 9-inch baking dish with olive oil.
Pierce the sweet potato and butternut squash with a fork and place in the oven. Bake for 45 minutes to an hour, until soft. Remove from the oven, let cool, and mash together, discarding the peel and seeds of the vegetables.
Spray a nonstick skillet with olive oil and heat over low heat. Add the chiles, garlic, onion, and ginger. Cook, stirring frequently, until the onions are soft, about 5 minutes. Add the greens, stirring thoroughly to mix with the ginger. Add the cumin and a pinch of salt. Cook until the greens wilt. Remove from the heat and let cool. When cool, squeeze as much extra fluid out as you can.

Lightly whip the egg whites, add the mashed tofu, and mix into the greens.

Combine the sweet potato mixture with the chopped walnuts and flaxseed.

Cut the phyllo sheets to conform to the size of the baking dish. Work with one sheet at a time and cover the rest with a damp towel. Spread the phyllo sheet flat on the bottom of the pan and spray lightly with olive oil. Continue with three more layers of dough.

Spread the greens mixture over the phyllo dough, then layer with three more layers of dough. Spread with the sweet potato mixture next, top with more layers of dough, then spread with the cottage cheese. Top with the final three layers of dough. Spray the top with olive oil.

Place on the middle shelf in the oven and bake at 350°F for 45 minutes.

Spanakopita, Spinach Pie

Calories per serving: 464
Percent of calories from:
Protein: 33
Carbohydrate: 40
Total fiber: 13 gm
Total cholesterol: 58 mg

Total fat: 14 g
%Saturated: 11
%Monounsaturated: 13
%Polyunsaturated: 106

Nutritional Profile:
percent of RDA per serving:
Vitamin A: 723
Vitamin C: 160
Vitamin E: 95
Vitamin B$_{12}$: 44
Iron: 95
Calcium: 61
Selenium: 75
Zinc: 40

GLOSSARY

alpha—Brain wave frequency indicative of a relaxed yet alert and re-flective state. Brain wave frequencies are rhythmic fluctuations of voltage between parts of the brain resulting in a flow of electric current that can be monitored by an electro-encephalograph (EEG).

amino acids—Small nitrogen-containing chemical units that link to-gether to form **protein** molecules. The body can make some of the amino acids it needs to construct its proteins, but others must be obtained from the diet.

anorexia nervosa—Psychological disorder in which the afflicted per-son intentionally consumes dangerously low quantities of food be-cause of a belief that it will improve his/her appearance or well-being. If untreated, can lead to death from malnutrition or from other complications. (See **bulimia.**) This is *not* a longevity diet! (See table 3.1 on page 45 for more on the differences between CR and anorexia nervosa.)

antiaging medicine—Type of medicine practiced by health-care pro-fessionals who seek to slow and, where possible, reverse the aging process of their patients. (See **life extension** and **geriatrics.**)

antioxidants—Molecules such as vitamins C and E (and even food additives such as BHT and BHA) that "mop up" or neutralize **free radicals.**

autoantibody—*Antibodies* are proteins produced by the immune system that bind to and neutralize or help neutralize substances thought to be germs or anything else that doesn't belong in the body. *Autoantibodies* are antibodies that target and bind to normally functioning parts of the body itself, thus causing diseases known as *autoimmune diseases*.

average life span—Average age of death of a group of organisms, be it a group of organisms in a scientific experiment or a group found in nature. (See **maximum life span.**)

biomarker—Indicator of some aspect of your state of health. Some biomarkers are simple, such as your pulse rate or the length of time you can balance on one foot with your eyes closed. Others are more sophisticated, for example, tests of substances found in your blood, such as cholesterol or fasting glucose. (See page 106 for a fuller discussion.)

BMI (Body Mass Index)—Measure of thinness or fatness that takes into account height.

Some people (who, for example, are very tall) would not be overweight if they weighed 190 pounds. A very short person who weighed 190 pounds would, on the other hand, almost certainly be overweight. BMI makes it easier to distinguish between those two types of people.

Specifically, BMI is calculated as your weight in kilograms divided by the square of your height in meters. The formula for BMI using height and weight in pounds and inches respectively is: 703 multiplied by weight in pounds divided by the square of height in inches. For example, if you weigh 170 pounds and are 5'9" (69 inches) tall, your BMI is 170 divided by 69, which is 25.1.

Note: Although BMI is a better measure of fitness than weight alone, it is still not perfect, since a flabby 190 pounds on someone with thin bones who was six feet tall would be far less healthy than a muscular 190 pounds on a person of the same height with a heavy bone structure.

bulimia—Psychological disorder related to anorexia nervosa in which the afflicted individual at times eats too little for good health, just as in anorexia, and at other times eats normal amounts of food (or perhaps even too much), but then forces him- or herself to vomit or in some other way—for example, manic, compulsive exercise or even laxative abuse—"get rid of" the consumed food that is perceived to have been excessive. The classic, clinical pattern of bulimia is a binge-and-purge cycle. (See **anorexia nervosa.**)

caloric allotment (**daily caloric allotment**)—Number of calories someone on CR allows him- or herself each day. For a large person on moderate CR, this might be as high as 2,500 or so, for a small person on a very extreme CR program, it might be under 1,500.

calorie—Unit of energy often used to measure the amount of energy in food. A calorie (not capitalized) is, technically, the amount of energy (or heat) needed to raise 1 gram of water by 1 degree Celsius (1.8 degrees Fahrenheit). The word *calorie,* when used to refer to the energy content of food, is actually a kilocalorie, or one thousand calories. Sometimes this food calorie is capitalized, "Calorie," to distinguish it from the other calorie. In this book, when we use "calorie," we mean kilocalorie.

control group—In a scientific experiment testing the effect of a medicine, dietary regimen, lifestyle change, or any other variable, at least two groups of laboratory animals (or people or plants or whatever is being tested) are needed: (1) the group on which the medicine or regimen is tested and (2) a group that doesn't take the medicine or undergo any other changes. The first group is called the **experimental group,** and the second is called the *control group.* The control group makes it possible to attribute changes in health observed in the experimental group to the intervention being tested, since everything else between the two groups was the same (that is, was "controlled").

CR Society International (**Calorie Restriction Society International**)—Nonprofit organization dedicated to helping people learn about and practice longevity diets, helping further CR research, and advancing the cause of antiaging medicine in general. (See Resources.)

dietary fiber—Plant material built up from simple sugars. The human body can derive no energy from fiber because we, unlike cows and many other animals, lack the enzymes needed to break down the fiber into its component sugars.

energy density—Measure of the amount of energy (or number of calories) in a given volume of food.

epidemiological evidence—Scientific evidence based on assessments of the disease patterns and health observed in relatively large populations.

epidemiology—Study of disease patterns in (generally large) human populations.

experimental group—(See **control group.**)

fatty acid—Type of lipid. Fatty acids are relatively small molecules that usually consist simply of a chain of carbon atoms with a *carboxylic acid group* (a carbon atom and an oxygen atom joined to an oxygen atom and a hydrogen atom, often represented as "COOH") at the end.

fiber—(See **dietary fiber.**)

free radicals—Highly reactive chemical fragments that can cause damage to vital molecules with which they come into contact. Free radicals are highly reactive because they contain unpaired electrons, which results in their "stealing" electrons from nearby molecules.

geriatrician—Physician whose specialty is **geriatrics,** that is, a physician who treats the elderly.

geriatrics—Medical specialty focused on the care of the elderly. (See **antiaging medicine.**)

gerontologist (or **research gerontologist**)—Scientist who studies the biology of aging.

gerontology—Scientific study of the biology of aging.

GI—(See **glycemic index.**)

glucose—Simple sugar that is the body's main source of fuel.

glycemic index (GI)—Measurement of the extent to which a food raises blood glucose levels. Pure glucose is arbitrarily assigned the reference value of 100. Foods with a GI below around 45 are considered **low-GI** foods; those with a GI above 70 or so are considered **high-GI** foods.

HDL (high-density lipoprotein)—Form of cholesterol that is thought to be healthful in part because it transports excess cholesterol to the liver, where it is eliminated. HDLs are often referred to as the "good cholesterol."

high-GI—(See **glycemic index.**)

homeostasis—Homeostasis is the physiological process by which various bodily systems (temperature, blood pressure, etc.) are maintained in a state of equilibrium, despite varying external conditions.

hydrogenation—Addition of hydrogen molecules to an unsaturated fatty acid such that it becomes more saturated. This is a process generally applied to vegetable oils (liquids), which turns them into fats (solids). The process is also referred to as "hardening." The fatty acids that result from this process are **trans-fatty acids.**

IGF-1 (Insulin-Like Growth Factor)—A hormone with many roles in the body. It assists with growth and development early in life, yet lower levels of the hormone later in life seem to be associated with slowed aging in many species. CR may exert its effects by lowering the level of IFG-1 in the blood and/or by lowering the extent to which IGF-1 can exert its effects.

LDL (low-density lipoprotein)—Form of cholesterol that contributes to the formation of plaque in the walls of arteries. It is often referred to as the "bad cholesterol."

life extension—Attempt to slow down and reverse the aging process. (See **antiaging medicine.**)

life span—Length of life of an organism. (See **average life span** and **maximum life span.**)

life-span study—Type of scientific study that measures the age of death of animals or subjects in a study, with the aim of determining which factors led to variations in mortality.

lipids—Very broad, diverse category of compounds, including fats, oils, steroids, waxes, that are generally insoluble in water. (See page 52 for a thorough discussion.)

low-GI—(See **glycemic index.**)

maximum life span—Length of life of the longest-lived member of a given species. For statistical reasons, maximum life span in experimental studies of antiaging interventions is sometimes measured not as the longest-lived member, but rather as the average of the longest-lived 10 percent, or 5 percent, and so on. (See **average life span.**)

minerals—In the context of nutrition: inorganic substances of (ultimately) nonbiologic origin that are essential for health.

monounsaturated fatty acid (MUFA)—Type of **fatty acid** with a chain of carbon atoms that is surrounded by ("saturated" with) hydrogen atoms except for just one "hole," or "unsaturated" spot, along the carbon chain. There is only one common dietary monounsaturated fatty acid, *oleic acid,* which is the primary constituent of olive oil and canola oil and is present in high quantities in avocados and many nuts.

MUFA—(See **monounsaturated fatty acid.**)

omega-3—Type of **polyunsaturated fatty acid** found in some nuts (for example, walnuts) and seeds (for example, flaxseeds) and, abundantly, in many coldwater fish such as salmon, with its first double bond (or "unsaturated spot") between the third and fourth carbon atoms from the *omega end* (also known as the *methyl end*) of the molecule.

omega-6—Type of **polyunsaturated fatty acid** like the *omega-3* fatty acids, except with the first double bond between the sixth and seventh carbon atoms from the omega end.

osteoporosis—Disease characterized by loss of calcium in bones, which results in bone brittleness and which leads to increased risk of fracture.

Oxygen Radical Absorbance Capacity (ORAC)—Test tube analysis that measures the total antioxidant power of foods.

phytochemicals—Literally: "plant chemical." Many of the hundreds that have been studied are thought to confer health benefits to those who consume them. Sometimes called *phytonutrients,* especially where a health role for a phytochemical has been solidly established.

phytonutrients—(See **phytochemicals.**)

polyunsaturated fatty acid (PUFA)—Type of **fatty acid** with a chain of carbon atoms that is surrounded by, or "saturated" with, hydrogen atoms, except for several "holes," or "unsaturated" spots, along the carbon chain. (If there is only one unsaturated spot along the chain, the fatty acid is a *monounsaturated fatty acid*.)

prospective study (sometimes called *cohort study*)—Type of scientific study in which certain independent variables such as caloric intake or exercise are measured at the beginning of the study, then the changes hypothesized to result from the independent variables are examined (longevity, incidence of cancer, diabetes, etc.). (See **retrospective study**.)

protein—Structurally and physiologically vital molecule, built up from smaller, nitrogen-rich chemical units known as **amino acids,** with multiple roles in essentially all life forms.

PUFA—(See **polyunsaturated fatty acid**.)

RDA (recommended daily allowance)—Widely used quantification, developed by the Food and Nutrition Board (a part of the National Academy of the Sciences), of the amount of each particular essential nutrient that the vast majority of healthy Americans (and others) should consume each day. Started being replaced by a more accurate set of several measurements, the dietary reference intakes (DRI), in the mid-1990s.

resveratrol—Small chemical produced by certain plants such as grape plants, partly as a defense against mold. Thought by many researchers to have a variety of health benefits. May be able to produce effects similar to calorie restriction (though much more research is needed).

retrospective study (sometimes called *case-control study*)—Type of scientific study in which a group with a certain preexisting disease or condition is compared with a group (the control group) without the affliction to discover what factors in the groups' respective histories might account for the difference in health between the groups. It is because researchers conducting this type of study are looking at the histories of the two groups that this kind of study is called *retrospective*. (See **prospective study**.)

saturated fatty acid—Type of **fatty acid** with a chain of carbon atoms that is entirely surrounded by ("saturated" with) hydrogen atoms. Common saturated fatty acids are solid at room temperature, as opposed to *unsaturated fatty acids* (both **polyunsaturated fatty acids** and **monounsaturated fatty acids**).

segmental aging—Name for the notion that different parts of the organism (different "segments") age at different rates. Some biomarkers might only measure the state of health or agedness of one or a few segments, not the whole organism. For example, one can have very high blood pressure, but very low fasting glucose.

set point—Weight your body "defends" when you are a young adult. That is, the weight your body tends toward if you make no special effort to lose or gain weight and don't exercise extraordinarily much or extraordinarily little. (See page 102 for a thorough discussion.)

trans-fatty acids—**Fatty acid** with two particular hydrogen atoms linked to the adjoining carbon atoms in a double bond and positioned farther away from each than in the nearly identical *cis* fatty acid, which is the form found much more often in nature. The *trans* form has a relatively straight molecular configuration, which makes it solid at room temperature. Trans-fatty acids exist in nature, but the overwhelming majority of the trans-fatty acid we consume was created by the **hydrogenation** process. This form of fatty acid is known to increase the risk for heart disease and may damage health in other ways as well.

vitamins—Molecules that cannot be manufactured by the body and are essential for health. (Literally, "vital amine.")

youth span—Period of time during which the state of health of an organism is youthful.

RESOURCES

ORGANIZATIONS SUPPORTING CR AND
RELATED LONGEVITY DIETS

Calorie Restriction Society International
(CR Society International)
The Calorie Restriction Society International
187 Ocean Drive
Newport, North Carolina 28570
USA
1-877-511-2702
http://www.crsociety.org

The CR Society is a nonprofit educational organization dedicated to teaching people about the Longevity Diet, supporting research into understanding how CR works and how it can best be implemented in humans, and critically exploring other health regimens that purport to offer similar benefits.

The CR Society is an essential resource for anyone interested in the Longevity Diet and, indeed, is an important resource for anyone interested in health in general.

Changing your life takes work. A support group is an essential resource. The CR Society's Internet-based discussion forums, as well as its growing number of regional support groups that have regular meetings, provide essential support and guidance to those interested in trying rigorous versions of the Longevity Diet.

The discussion forums also provide an easy way to get feedback on your own longevity program from experienced practitioners of the Longevity Diet. No one book can speak to all the particular issues that each reader would want addressed. But among the 1,500 (and growing) members, you will likely find someone facing challenges similar to those you are facing.

In addition, because the group was founded by "life extensionists"—those interested in slowing the aging process and living very, *very* long, healthy lives—there is a constant engagement with cutting-edge biological research. When relevant new research findings appear that could affect your health, you will probably hear about these findings first via the CR Society.

Membership in the CR Society includes many other benefits, a newsletter, discounts at our conferences, and more, which you can read about at the above Web site.

Walford Web Site
http://www.walford.com

Roy Walford's Web site contains pointers to a great number of resources for people interested in living longer, healthier lives. In addition, there is a lot of historical information about Roy Walford's extraordinary life. Take a look at this Web site if you simply want to get inspired about life and its many possibilities!

Dr. Walford's Interactive Diet Planner
http://www.walford.com

Popularly known as DWIDP, this software program is a helpful companion to this book. Using the U.S. Department of Agriculture database of over six thousand foods, including whole, name brand, processed, and fast foods, it is designed to allow you to put together optimal daily or weekly food combinations to achieve the highest quality and full RDA values at the lowest calorie intake. The unique powerhouse of DWIDP, not found like this in any other nutrition software program, is the Search Engine. It works like this: suppose you are on a 1,600-calorie diet and today's food list comes to 1,200 calories, 25 percent derived from fat, and DWIDP tells you the RDAs for selenium, vitamin B_6, and calcium are low. What single food or two foods can you add, 400 calories of which will make up the difference, and also be low in fat? DWIDP will tell you this or any other combination of desires, and no other program will. You can maximize, minimize, or optimize one or many items, and at the same time. Twenty-eight nutrients are covered in the program. A Tutorial and Help program guide you through the interactive capabilities of DWIDP. Up to ninety-nine users may each have a personal profile based on height, age, frame size, and desired percentage of fat.

NutriBase Nutrition Software
http://www.nutribase.com

NutriBase is a nutrition software program with enough features to satisfy any techie, yet its graphical interface makes navigation fairly easy and user friendly for home use. NutriBase uses the USDA R14 nutrient database as well as name-brand and restaurant entries and features over thirty-one thousand food entries. Depending on which of the home-use versions you choose, you can select from fifty-one to eighty-eight nutrients to monitor. You can specify which nutrients you wish to use in your analysis, thus customizing your reports. It is easy to find the foods you need, and you can organize your recipes into twenty-six folders.

You can customize your toolbar and easily resize or resequence columns of data for ease of use. You can also view meals, recipes, and foods in a spreadsheet that ranks them according to parameters that you select.

The fitness manager comes with all versions of NutriBase. Calorie expenditures are calculated according to your activity, and weight loss can be charted and predicted with the fitness manager.

The Personal Edition tracks alcohol, caffeine, and sugars, and the Personal Plus edition also tracks vitamins.

The home-user versions of NutriBase are extremely rewarding. The NutriBase Clinical edition is a high-end program that was named the official dietary monitoring software for the "Calorie Restriction with Optimal Nutrition Effects Pilot Study." It is the obvious choice for professionals in the nutrition, fitness, and health industries. The Clinical edition tracks minerals and omega fatty acids.

For more information on the home editions of NutriBase, please visit http://dietsoftware.com. For the professional version, visit http://www .nutribase.com.

Cronometer
http://spaz.ca/cronometer/

This is a free, open source and cross-platform diet software program. Along with the basics of tracking your nutritional profile over one or several days, preparing recipes, and sharing data and recipes, the Cronometer also allows you to track and chart your biometrics.

Nutrition Data.com
http://www.nutritiondata.com/tools/nutrient-search

This site allows you to search the USDA food database to find foods that are highest (or lowest) in particular nutrients. For instance, you could look for foods that are rich in calcium and low in calories.

NOTES

CHAPTER 1

1. U.S. Department of Agriculture, U.S. Department of Health and Human Services, *Dietary Guidelines for Americans*, 3rd ed., 1990. (*Home and Garden Bulletin*, no. 232.)

2. U.S. Department of Agriculture, U.S. Department of Health and Human Services, *Nutrition and Your Health: Dietary Guidelines for Americans*, 5th ed., 2000.

3. U.S. Department of Agriculture, U.S. Department of Health and Human Services, "New Dietary Guidelines Will Help Americans Make Better Food Choices, Live Healthier Lives." (Press release: www.hhs.gov/news/press/2005.html.) Emphasis on reducing calorie intake will also be part of the forthcoming 2010 edition of "Dietary Guidelines for Americans." See http://www.cnpp.usda.gov/DietaryGuidelines.htm. (Last accessed Saturday, January 07, 2010.)

4. Roy L. Walford, *Beyond the 120-Year Diet: How to Double Your Vital Years* (New York: Four Walls Eight Windows, 2000). Previously published in 1986 as *The 120-Year Diet*.

CHAPTER 2

1. http://www.nhlbi.nih.gov/health/public/heart/obesity/lose_wt/index.htm. (Last accessed November 06, 2009.)

2. E. B. Edney and R. W. Gill, "Evolution of Senescence and Specific Longevity," *Nature* 220, no. 164 (October 19, 1968): 281–82.

3. R. Weindruch, "Caloric Restriction and Aging," *Scientific American* 274, no. 1 (January 1996): 46–52.

4. S. N. Austad, "Life Extension by Dietary Restriction in the Bowl and Doily Spider, *Frontinella pyramitela*," *Experimental Gerontology* 24, no. 1 (1989): 83–92.

5. B. K. Patnaik, N. Mahapatro, and B. S. Jena, "Ageing in Fishes," *Gerontology* 40, nos. 2–4 (1994): 113–32.

6. M. H. Ross, "Length of Life and Caloric Intake," *The American Journal of Clinical Nutrition* 8 (August 25, 1972): 834–38.

7. Centers for Disease Control and Prevention, U.S. Department of Health and Human Services, *National Vital Statistics Reports*, 52, no. 9 (November 7, 2003).

8. R. L. Walford, D. Mock, R. Verdery, and T. MacCallum, "Calorie Restriction in Biosphere 2: Alterations in Physiologic, Hematologic, Hormonal, and Biochemical Parameters in Humans Restricted for a 2-Year Period," *The Journals of Gerontology. Series A, Biological Sciences and Medical Sciences* 57, no. 6 (June 2002): B211–24.

9. L. Fontana, T. E. Meyer, S. Klein, and J. O. Holloszy, "Long-term Calorie Restriction Is Highly Effective in Reducing the Risk for Atherosclerosis in Humans," *Proceedings of the National Academy of Sciences of the United States of America* 101, no. 17 (April 27, 2004): 6, 659–63.

10. R. L. Walford and R. Weindruch. *The Retardation of Aging and Disease by Dietary Restriction* (Springfield, IL: Thomas, 1988).

11. M. T. Goodman, J. H. Hankin, L. R. Wilkens, L. C. Lyu, K. McDuffie, L.Q. Liu, and L. N. Kolonel, "Diet, Body Size, Physical Activity, and the Risk of Endometrial Cancer," *Cancer Research* 57, no. 22 (November 15, 1997): 5077–85; A. S. Furberg and I. Thune, "Metabolic Abnormalities (Hypertension, Hyperglycemia and Overweight), Lifestyle (High Energy Intake and Physical Inactivity) and Endometrial Cancer Risk in a Norwegian Cohort," *Journal International du Cancer* 104, no. 6 (May 10, 2003): 669–76; A. Mellemgaard, J. K. McLaughlin, K. Overvad, and J. H. Olsen, "Dietary Risk Factors for Renal Cell Carcinoma in Denmark," *European Journal of Cancer* 32A, no. 4 (April 1996): 673–82.

12. N. Pitsikas, M. Carli, S. Fidecka, and S. Algeri, "Effect of Life-long Hypocaloric Diet on Age-Related Changes in Motor and Cognitive Behavior in a Rat Population," *Neurobiology of Aging* 11, no. 4 (July–Aug 1990): 417–23; C. L. Goodrick, "Effects of Lifelong Restricted Feeding on Complex Maze Performance in Rats," *AGE* 7:1–2.

13. L. W. Means, J. L. Higgins, and T. J. Fernandez, "Midlife Onset of Dietary Restriction Extends Life and Prolongs Cognitive Functioning," *Physiology & Behavior* 54, no. 3 (September 1993): 503–508; F. Idrobo, K. Nandy, D. I. Mostofsky, L. Blatt, and L. Nandy, "Dietary Restriction: Effects on Radial Maze Learning and Lipofuscin Pigment Deposition in the Hippocampus and Frontal Cortex," *Archives of Gerontology and Geriatrics* 6, no. 4 (December 1987): 355–62.

14. C. Moreschi, *Beziehungen zwischen Ernährung und Tumorwachsen* [The Connection Between Nutrition and Tumor Promotion], *Zeitschrift für Immunitätsforsch* 2 (1909): 651–75.

15. C. M. McCay, M. F. Crowel, and L. A. Maynard, "The Effect of Retarded Growth upon the Length of the Life Span and upon the Ultimate Body Size," *The Journal of Nutrition* 10 (1935): 63–79.

16. A. Koizumi, Y. Wada, M. Tuskada, T. Kayo, M. Naruse, K. Horiuchi, T. Mogi, M. Yoshioka, M. Sasaki, Y. Miyamaura, T. Abe, K. Ohtomo, and R. L. Walford, "A Tumor Preventive Effect of Dietary Restriction Is Antagonized by a High Housing Temperature through Deprivation of Torpor," *Mechanisms of Ageing and Development* 92, no. 1 (November 29, 1996): 67–82.

17. B. Conti, "Considerations on Temperature, Longevity and Aging," *Cellular and Molecular Life Sciences* 65, no. 11 (June 2008): 1626–30.

18. E. J. Masoro, "Antiaging Action of Caloric Restriction: Endocrine and Metabolic Aspects," *Obesity Research* 3, suppl. 2 (September 1995): 241s–47s.

19. S. R. Spindler, J. M. Grizzle, R. L. Walford, and P. L. Mote, "Aging and Restriction of Dietary Calories Increases Insulin Receptor mRNA, and Aging Increases Glucocorticoid Receptor mRNA in the Liver of Female C3B10RF1 Mice," *Journal of Gerontology* 46, no. 6 (November 1991): B233–37; B. C. Hansen, "Obesity, Diabetes, and Insulin Resistance: Implications from Molecular Biology, Epidemiology, and Experimental Studies in Humans and Animals," Synopsis of the American Diabetes Association's 29th Research Symposium and Satellite Conference of the 7th International Congress on Obesity, Boston, Massachusetts, *Diabetes Care* 18, no. 6 (June 1995): A2–9.

20. G. S. Roth, M. A. Lane, D. K. Ingram, J. A. Mattison, D. Elahi, J. D. Tobin, D. Muller, and E. J. Metter, "Biomarkers of Caloric Restriction May Predict Longevity in Humans," *Science* 297 (2002): 811.

21. T. A. Hughes, J. T. Gwynne, B. R. Switzer, C. Herbst, and G. White, "Effects of Caloric Restriction and Weight Loss on Glycemic

Control, Insulin Release and Resistance, and Atherosclerotic Risk in Obese Patients with Type II Diabetes Mellitus," *The American Journal of Medicine* 77, no. 1 (July 1984): 7–17; R. I. Misbin, "Dietary Regulation of Insulin Receptors in Obesity," *The Journal of Nutrition* 111, no. 3 (March 1981): 475–79; P. J. Savage, L. J. Bennion, and P. H. Bennett, "Normalization of Insulin and Glucagon Secretion in Ketosis-Resistant Diabetes Mellitus with Prolonged Diet Therapy," *The Journal of Clinical Endocrinology and Metabolism* 49, no. 6 (December 1979): 830–33.

22. American Diabetes Association, "Evidence-Based Nutrition Principles and Recommendations for the Treatment and Prevention of Diabetes and Related Complications," *Diabetes Care* 25 (2002): S50–60.

23. J. O. Holloszy and L Fontana, "Caloric Restriction in Humans," *Experimental Gerontology* 42, no. 8 (August 2007): 709–12.

24. J. M. Lipman, A. Turturro, and R. W. Hart, "The Influence of Dietary Restriction on DNA Repair in Rodents: A Preliminary Study," *Mechanisms of Ageing and Development* 48, no. 2 (May 1989): 135–43.

25. R. S. Sohal, S. Agarwal, M. Candas, M. J. Forster, and H. Lal, "Effect of Age and Caloric Restriction on DNA Oxidative Damage in Different Tissues of C57BL/6 Mice," *Mechanisms of Ageing and Development* 76, nos. 2–3 (October 20, 1994): 215–24; V. Haley-Zitlin and A. Richardson, "Effect of Dietary Restriction on DNA Repair and DNA Damage," *Mutation Research* 295, nos. 4–6 (December 1993): 237–45.

26. C. M. Gedik, G. Grant, P. C. Morrice, S. G Wood, and A. R. Collins, "Effects of Age and Dietary Restriction on Oxidative DNA Damage, Antioxidant Protection and DNA Repair in Rats," *European Journal of Nutrition* (July 28, 2004); D. C. Cabelof, S. Yanamadala, J. J. Raffoul, Z. Guo, A. Soofi, and A. R. Heydari, "Caloric Restriction Promotes Genomic Stability by Induction of Base Excision Repair and Reversal of Its Age-Related Decline," *DNA Repair* 2, no. 3 (March 1, 2003): 295–307.

27. T. Hofer, L. Fontana, S. D. Anton, E. P. Weiss, D. Villareal, B. Malayappan, and C. Leeuwenburgh, "Long-Term Effects of Caloric Restriction or Exercise on DNA and RNA Oxidation Levels in White Blood Cells and Urine in Humans," *Rejuvenation Research* 11, no. 4 (August 2008): 793–99.

28. N. J. O'Callaghan, P. M. Clifton, M. Noakes, and M. Fenech, "Weight Loss in Obese Men Is Associated with Increased Telomere

Length and Decreased Abasic Sites in Rectal Mucosa," *Rejuvenation Research* 12, no. 3 (June 2009):169–76.

29. D. Kritchevsky, "Caloric Restriction and Cancer," *Journal of Nutritional Science and Vitaminology* 47, no. 1 (February 2001): 13–19; S. D. Hursting and F. W. Kari, "The Anticarcinogenic Effects of Dietary Restriction: Mechanisms and Future Directions," *Mutation Research* 43, nos. 1–2 (July 15, 1999): 235–49; B. S. Hass, R. W. Hart, M. H. Lu, and B. D. Lyn-Cook, "Effects of Caloric Restriction in Animals on Cellular Function, Oncogene Expression, and DNA Methylation in Vitro," *Mutation Research* 295, nos. 4–6 (December 1993): 281–89.

30. See, for example, K. B. Michels, A. Ekbom, "Caloric Restriction and Incidence of Breast Cancer," *JAMA: The Journal of the American Medical Association* 291, no. 10 (March 10, 2004): 1, 226–30; F. C. Papadopoulos, I. Pantziaras, P. Lagiou, L. Brandt, L. Ekselius, and A. Ekbom, "Age at Onset of Anorexia Nervosa and Breast Cancer Risk," *European Journal of Cancer Prevention* 18, no. 3 (June 2009): 207–11.

31. A. M. Holehan and B. J. Merry, "Modification of the Oestrous Cycle Hormonal Profile by Dietary Restriction," *Mechanisms of Ageing and Development* 32, no. 1 (October 14, 1985): 63–76.

32. C. J. Carr, J. T. King, and M. B. Visscher, "The Effects of Dietary Caloric Restriction on Maturity and Senescence, with Particular Reference to Fertility and Longevity," *The American Journal of Physiology* 15 (1947): 511–19.

33. Roy L. Walford, *Maximum Life Span* (New York: Norton, 1983): 90.

34. J. F. Nelson, R. G. Gosden, and L. S. Felicio, "Effect of Dietary Restriction on Estrous Cyclicity and Follicular Reserves in Aging C57BL/6J Mice," *Biology of Reproduction* 32, no. 3 (April 1985): 515–22.

35. For a review, see H. Y. Chung, B. Sung, K. J. Jung, Y. Zou, and B. P. Yu, "The Molecular Inflammatory Process in Aging," *Antioxidants & Redox Signaling* 8, nos. 3–4 (March–April 2006): 572–81.

36. A. Hiona and C. Leeuwenburgh, "Effects of Age and Caloric Restriction on Brain Neuronal Cell Death/Survival," *Annals of the New York Academy of Sciences* (June 2004) 1019: 96–105.

37. L. Fontana, T. E. Meyer, S. Klein, J. O. Holloszy, "Long-term Calorie Restriction Is Highly Effective in Reducing the Risk for Atherosclerosis in Humans," *Proceedings of the National Academy of Sciences of the United States of America* 101, no. 17 (April 27, 2004): 6, 659–63.

CHAPTER 3

1. From an interview quoted by Reuters. Study: "Special Diets Don't Mean More Weight Loss." Reuters newsfeed (via www.yahoo.com), November 9, 2004. The research was reported in M. L. Dansinger, J. L. Gleason, and J. L. Griffith, et al., "One-Year Effectiveness of the Atkins, Ornish, Weight Watchers, and Zone Diets in Decreasing Body Weight and Heart Disease Risk," presented at the American Heart Association Scientific Sessions, November 12, 2003, in Orlando, FL.

2. R. B. Ervin, J. D. Wright, C. Y. Wang, and J. Kennedy-Stephenson, "Dietary Intake of Fats and Fatty Acids for the United States Population: 1999–2000," *Advance Data* 348 (November 8, 2004): 1–6.

3. B. R. Hammond Jr., E. J. Johnson, R. M. Russell, N. I. Krinsky, K. J. Yeum, R. B. Edwards, and D. M. Snodderly, "Dietary Modification of Human Macular Pigment Density," *Investigative Ophthalmology & Visual Science* 38, no. 9 (August 1997): 1,795–801.

4. J. K. Campbell, K. Canene-Adams, B. L. Lindshield, T. W. Boileau, S. K. Clinton, and J. W. Erdman Jr., "Tomato Phytochemicals and Prostate Cancer Risk," *The Journal of Nutrition* 134, suppl. 12 (December 2004): 3486S–92S.

5. E. R. Miller III, R. Pastor-Barriuso, D. Dalal, R. A. Riemersma, L. J. Appel, and E. Guallar, "Meta-Analysis: High-Dosage Vitamin E Supplementation May Increase All-Cause Mortality," *Annals of Internal Medicine* 142, no. 1 (January 4, 2005): 37–46. Note: The authors of the paper acknowledge several limitations to their analysis, the most important of which is that the studies that involved very high doses of vitamin E were often very small, and were conducted on patients with chronic illnesses.

6. Katherine Tallmadge, "Eat Less, Live Longer?" *The Washington Post* (May 19, 2004): F1.

CHAPTER 4

1. http://csde.washington.edu/downloads/01–04.pdf.

2. A. Salminen and K. Kaarniranta, "Insulin/IGF-1 Paradox of Aging: Regulation via AKT/IKK/NF-kappaB Signaling," *Cellular Signalling* (October 26, 2009).

3. J. A. Mattison, M. A. Lane, G. S. Roth, and D. K. Ingram, "Calorie Restriction in Rhesus Monkeys," *Experimental Gerontology* 38, nos. 1–2 (January–February 2003): 35–46.

4. R. L. Walford, D. Mock, R. Verdery, and T. MacCallum, "Calorie Restriction in Biosphere 2: Alterations in Physiologic, Hematologic,

Hormonal, and Biochemical Parameters in Humans Restricted for a 2-Year Period," *The Journals of Gerontology. Series A, Biological Sciences and Medical Sciences* 57, no. 6 (June 2002): B211–24; L. M. Redman, C. K. Martin, D. A. Williamson, and E. Ravussin, "Effect of Caloric Restriction in Non-Obese Humans on Physiological, Psychological and Behavioral Outcomes," *Physiology & Behavior* 94, no. 5 (August 6, 2008): 643–648; L. M. Redman and E. Ravussin, "Endocrine Alterations in Response to Calorie Restriction in Humans," *Molecular and Cellular Endocrinology* 299, no. 1 (February 5, 2009): 129–36.

5. W. R. Pendergrass, P. E. Penn, J. Li, and N. S. Wolf, "Age-Related Telomere Shortening in Lens Epithelium From Old Rats Is Slowed by Caloric Restriction," *Experimental Eye Research* 73, no. 2 (August 2001): 221–28.

6. While there are plenty of reasons to keep your fasting glucose levels low, and although the glycemic theory of aging is intuitively appealing, one recent study suggests that glucose may actually be a less important part of the CR effect than previously thought. The study compared four groups of mice, one with a gene causing altered glucose levels, placed on CR; another with that same gene but not placed on CR; and then two groups without the gene, again one group on CR, one not. Survival was associated with degree of CR, not with circulating glucose levels. However, this was only one study, as of yet not repeated. See R. McCarter, W. Mejia, Y. Ikeno, V. Monnier, K. Kewitt, M. Gibbs, A. McMahan, and R. Strong, "Plasma Glucose and the Action of Calorie Restriction on Aging," *The Journals of Gerontology. Series A, Biological Sciences and Medical Sciences* 62, no. 10 (October 2007): 1059–70.

7. M. Barbieri, M. R. Rizzo, D. Manzella, R. Grella, E. Ragno, M. Carbonella, A. M. Abbatecola, and G. Paolisso, "Glucose Regulation and Oxidative Stress in Healthy Centenarians," *Experimental Gerontology* 38, nos. 1–2 (January–February 2003): 137–43.

8. N. Libina, J. Berman, and C. Kenyon, "Tissue-Specific Activities of *C. elegans* DAF-16 in the Regulation of Life Span," *Cell* 115, no. 4:489–502; M. Tatar, "The Neuroendocrine Regulation of Drosophila Aging," *Experimental Gerontology* 39, nos. 11–12 (November 2004): 1745–50.

9. G. Bjelakovic, D. Nikolova, L.L. Gluud, R.G. Simonetti, and C. Gluud, "Mortality in Randomized Trials of Antioxidant Supplements for Primary and Secondary Prevention: Systematic Review and Meta-

Analysis," *Journal of the American Medical Association* 297 (2007): 842–57.

10. M. Ristow, K. Zarse, A. Oberbach, N. Klöting, M. Birringer, M. Kiehntopf, M. Stumvoll, C.R. Kahn, and M. Blüher, "Antioxidants Prevent Health-Promoting Effects of Physical Exercise in Humans," *Proceedings of the National Academy of Sciences of the United States of America* 106, no. 21 (May 26, 2009): 8665–70.

11. R. Gredilla, A. Sanz, M. Lopez-Torres, and G. Barja, "Caloric Restriction Decreases Mitochondrial Free Radical Generation at Complex I and Lowers Oxidative Damage to Mitochondrial DNA in the Rat Heart," *The FASEB Journal: Official Publication of the Federation of American Societies for Experimental Biology* 15, no. 9 (July 2001): 1589–91.

12. S. X. Cao, J. M. Dhahbi, P. L. Mote, and S. R. Spindler, "Genomic Profiling of Short- and Long-Term Caloric Restriction Effects in the Liver of Aging Mice," *Proceedings of the National Academy of Sciences of the United States of America* 98, no. 19 (September 11, 2001): 10630–35.

13. R. J. Colman, T. M. Beasley, D. B. Allison, and R. Weindruch, "Attenuation of Sarcopenia By Dietary Restriction in Rhesus Monkeys," *The Journals of Gerontology. Series A, Biological Sciences and Medical Sciences* 63, no. 6 (June 2008): 556–59.

14. R. J. Colman, R. M. Anderson, S. C. Johnson, E. K. Kastman, K. J. Kosmatka, T. M. Beasley, D. B. Allison, C. Cruzen, H. A. Simmons, J. W. Kemnitz, and R. Weindruch, "Caloric Restriction Delays Disease Onset and Mortality in Rhesus Monkeys," *Science* 325, no. 5937 (July 10, 2009): 201–204.

15. N. L. Bodkin, T. M. Alexander, H. K. Ortmeyer, E. Johnson, and B. C. Hansen, "Mortality and Morbidity in Laboratory-Maintained Rhesus Monkeys and Effects of Long-Term Dietary Restriction," *The Journals of Gerontology. Series A, Biological Sciences and Medical Sciences* 58, no. 3 (March 2003): 212–19.

16. R. J. Coleman, et al.

17. T. E. Meyer, S. J. Kovács, A. A. Ehsani, S. Klein, J. O. Holloszy, and L. Fontana, "Long-Term Caloric Restriction Ameliorates the Decline in Diastolic Function in Humans," *Journal of the American College of Cardiology* 47, no. 2 (January 17, 2006): 398–402.

18. M. M. Riordan, E. P. Weiss, T. E. Meyer, A. A. Ehsani, S. B. Racette, D. T. Villareal, L. Fontana, J. O. Holloszy, and S. J. Kovács, "The Effects of Caloric Restriction and Exercise-Induced Weight Loss on Left

Ventricular Diastolic Function," *American Journal of Physiology. Heart and Circulatory Physiology* 294, no. 3 (March 2008): H1174–82.

19. T. Hofer, L. Fontana, S. D. Anton, E. P. Weiss, D. Villareal, B. Malayappan, and C. Leeuwenburgh, "Long-Term Effects of Caloric Restriction or Exercise on DNA and RNA Oxidation Levels in White Blood Cells and Urine in Humans," *Rejuvenation Research* 11, no. 4 (August 2008): 793–99.

20. J. O. Holloszy, and L. Fontana, "Caloric Restriction in Humans," *Experimental Gerontology* 42, no. 8 (August 2007): 709–12.

21. L. Fontana, E. P. Weiss, D. T. Villareal, S. Klein, and J. O. Holloszy, "Long-Term Effects of Calorie or Protein Restriction on Serum IGF-1 and IGFBP-3 Concentration in Humans," *Aging Cell* 7, no. 5 (October 2008): 681–87.

22. Spindler.

23. J. G. Wood, B. Rogina, S. Lavu, K. Howitz, S. L. Helfand, M. Tatar, and D. Sinclair, "Sirtuin Activators Mimic Caloric Restriction and Delay Aging in Metazoans," *Nature* 430, no. 7000 (August 5, 2004): 686–89; S. Jarolim, J. Millen, G. Heeren, P. Laun, D. S. Goldfarb, and M. Breitenbach, "A Novel Assay for Replicative Lifespan in *Saccharomyces Cerevisiae*," *FEMS Yeast Research* 5 no. 2 (November 2004): 169–77.

24. M. Kaeberlein, T. McDonagh, B. Heltweg, J. Hixon, E. A. Westman, S. Caldwell, A. Napper, R. Curtis, P. S. Distefano, S. Fields, A. Bedalov, and B. K. Kennedy, "Substrate Specific Activation of Sirtuins by Resveratrol," *The Journal of Biological Chemistry* (January 31, 2005).

25. J. A. Baur, K. J. Pearson, N. L. Price, H. A. Jamieson, C. Lerin, A. Kalra, V. V. Prabhu, J. S. Allard, G. Lopez-Lluch, K. Lewis, P. J. Pistell, S. Poosala, K. G. Becker, O. Boss, D. Gwinn, M. Wang, S. Ramaswamy, K. W. Fishbein, R. G. Spencer, E. G. Lakatta, D. Le Couteur, R. J. Shaw, P. Navas, P. Puigserver, D. K. Ingram, R. de Cabo, and D. A. Sinclair, "Resveratrol Improves Health and Survival of Mice on a High-Calorie Diet," *Nature* 444, no. 7117 (November 16, 2006): 337–42.

26. J. L. Barger, T. Kayo, J. M. Vann, E. B. Arias, J. Wang, T. A. Hacker, Y. Wang, D. Raederstorff, J. D. Morrow, C. Leeuwenburgh, D. B. Allison, K. W. Saupe, G. D. Cartee, R. Weindruch, and T. A. Prolla, "A Low Dose of Dietary Resveratrol Partially Mimics Caloric Restriction and Retards Aging Parameters in Mice," *PLoS One* 3, no. 6 (June 4, 2008): e2264.

27. D. E. Harrison, R. Strong, Z. D. Sharp, J. F. Nelson, C. M. Astle, K. Flurkey, N. L. Nadon, J. E. Wilkinson, K. Frenkel, C. S. Carter, M. Pahor, M. A. Javors, E. Fernandez, and R. A. Miller, "Rapamycin Fed

Late in Life Extends Lifespan in Genetically Heterogeneous Mice," *Nature* 460, no. 7253 (July 16, 2009): 392–95.

CHAPTER 5
1. Ch. Barrows Jr. and L. M. Roeder, "The Effect of Reduced Dietary Intake on Enzymatic Activities and Life Span of Rats," *Journal of Gerontology* 20 (January 1965): 69–71.

CHAPTER 6
1. Sources include *The New England Journal of Medicine* (June 26, 2003); Dimitrios Trichopoulos, MD, PhD, professor of epidemiology; Vincent L. Gregory, professor of cancer prevention, Harvard School of Public Health, Boston; Alice H. Lichtenstein, DSc, senior scientist and director, Cardiovascular Nutrition Laboratory; Jean Mayer, USDA Human Nutrition Researcher Center on Aging, Tufts University, Boston; spokeswoman, American Heart Association.

2. J. A. Menendez, A. Vazquez-Martin, R. Garcia-Villalba, A. Carrasco-Pancorbo, C. Oliveras-Ferraros, A. Fernandez-Gutierrez, and A. Segura-Carretero, "Anti-HER2 (erbB-2) Oncogene Effects of Phenolic Compounds Directly Isolated from Commercial Extra-Virgin Olive Oil (EVOO)," *BMC Cancer* 8 (December 18, 2008): 377.

3. "Olive Oil: A Cheap Bottle Beats a Pricier Lineup," *Consumer Reports* (September 2004).

4. B. Rolls and R. A. Barnett, *The Volumetrics Weight-Control Plan: Feel Full on Fewer Calories* (New York: HarperTorch, 2003).

CHAPTER 7
1. http://www.photosmash.net/Usda_data/foods_db.html, Author Karen McCann. Dr Walford's Food Database Access. (Last accessed October 31, 2009.)

2. http://spaz.ca/cronometer/ Author Aaron Davidson. (Last accessed October 31, 2009.)

3. http://www.nutritiondata.com/tools/nutrient-search, CondéNet. (Last accessed October 31, 2009.)

4. www.nal.usda.gov/fnic/foodcomp/search/index.html, United States Department of Agriculture, Agriculture Research Service. (Last accessed October 31, 2009.)

CHAPTER 10

1. E. T. Poehlman, A. Turturro, N. Bodkin, W. Cefalu, S. Heymsfield, J. Holloszy, and J. Kemnitz, "Caloric Restriction Mimetics, Physical Activity and Body Composition Changes," The Gerontological Society of America, 2001.

2. T. E. Meyer, S. J. Kovacs, A. A. Ehsani, S. Klein, J. O. Holloszy, and L. Fontana, "Long-Term Caloric Restriction Ameliorates the Decline in Diastolic Function in Humans," *Journal of the American College of Cardiology*, 47, no. 2 (January 17, 2006): 398–402.

3. R. Kalani, S. Judge, C. Carter, M. Pahor, and C. Leeuwenburgh, "Effects of Caloric Restriction and Exercise on Age-Related, Chronic Inflammation Assessed by C-Reactive Protein and Interleukin-6," *Journals of Gerontology* 61 (2006): 211–17.

4. L. K. Heilbronn, L. de Jonge, M. I. Frisard, J. P. DeLany, D. E. Larson-Meyer, J. Rood, T. Nguyen, C. K. Martin, J. Volaufova, M. M. Most, F. L. Greenway, S. R. Smith, W. A. Deutsch, D. A. Williamson, and E. Ravussin, "Effect of 6-Month Calorie Restriction on Biomarkers of Longevity, Metabolic Adaptation, and Oxidative Stress in Overweight Individuals," *Journal of the American Medical Association* 295 (2006): 1539–48.

5. S. J. Colcombe, A. F. Kramer, E. McAuley, K. I. Erickson, and P. Scalf, "Neurocognitive Aging and Cardiovascular Fitness: Recent Findings and Future Directions," *Journal of Molecular Neuroscience: MN* 24, no. 1 (2004): 9–14 (Review).

6. Svatmarama, *Hatha Yoga Pradipika*, commentary Hans-Ulrich Reiker (London: Aquarian Press, 1992).

7. J. A. Raub, "Psychophysiologic Effects of Hatha Yoga on Musculoskeletal and Cardiopulmonary Functions: A Literature Review," *Journal of Complementary and Alternative Medicine* 8 (2002): 797–812; C. H. Patel, "Yoga and Bio-feedback in the Management of Hypertension," *Lancet* 2, no. 837 (1973): 1053–55; S. B. Khalsa, "Treatment of Chronic Insomnia with Yoga: A Preliminary Study with Sleep-Wake Diaries," *Applied Psychophysiological Biofeedback* 29, no. 4 (December 2004): 269–78; K. A. Williams, J. Petronis, D. Smith, D. Goodrich, J. Wu, N. Ravi, E. J. Doyle Jr., R. Gregory Juckett, M. Munoz Kolar, R. Gross, and L. Steinberg, "Effect of Iyengar Yoga Therapy for Chronic Low Back Pain," *Pain* 115, nos. 1–2 (May 2005): 107–17.

8. K. J. Sherman, D. C. Cherkin, J. Erro, D. L. Miglioretti, and R. A. Deyo, "Comparing Yoga, Exercise, and a Self-Care Book for Chronic

Low Back Pain: A Randomized, Controlled Trial," *Annals of Internal* 143, no. 12 (December 20, 2005): 849–56; Williams et al.

9. D. Shapiro, I. A. Cook, D. M. Davydov, C. Ottaviani, A. F Leuchter, and M. Abrams, "Yoga as a Complementary Treatment of Depression: Effects of Traits and Moods on Treatment Outcome," *Evidence Based Complementary and Alternative Medicine* 4, no. 4 (December 2007): 493–502.

10. Khalsa.

11. M. S. Garfinkel, H. R. Schumacher Jr., A. Husain, M. Levy, and R. A. Reshetar, "Evaluation of a Yoga-Based Regimen for Treatment of Osteoarthritis of the Hands," *Journal of Rheumatology* 21, no. 12 (December 1994): 2341–43.

12. K. Khattab, A. A. Khattab, J. Ortak, G. Richardt, and H. Bonnemeier, "Iyengar Yoga Increases Cardiac Parasympathetic Nervous Modulation Among Healthy Yoga Practitioners," *Evidence Based Complementary and Alternative Medicine* 4, no. 4 (December 2007): 511–17.

13. Mel Robin, *A Physiological Handbook for Teachers of Yogasana* (Tucson: Fenestra Books, 2002), 271.

14. E. S. Epel and E. H. Blackburn at the University of California–San Francisco, as reported online www.pnas.org/cgi/content/abstract/0407162101v1 (last accessed: November 05, 2009) in *Proceedings of the National Academy of Sciences* (November 2004).

15. S. Sandberg, S. Jarvenpaa, A. Penttinen, J. Y. Paton, and D. C. McCann, "Asthma Exacerbations in Children Immediately Following Stressful Life Events: A Cox's Hierarchical Regression," *Thorax* 59, no. 12 (December 2004): 1046–51.

ACKNOWLEDGMENTS

This book owes its essence and its every word to the late Dr. Roy Lee Walford, friend to us both, father to Lisa, and mentor to Brian. Dr. Walford's work has given youth and life to tens of thousands and inspiration to us and to many others. We hope this book helps in some way to keep his spirit with us.

The authors also wish to acknowledge a debt to the untiring technical support of Ross R. Smith, who enabled us to collaborate despite only rarely being on the same continent. His wizardry with computers, wireless Internet connections, and Internet telephony proved invaluable. We are also grateful to the members of the CR Society International who, through their pioneering spirit, pushed the envelope of CR and shared their experiences with the rest of us, thus enabling us and many others to fine-tune our health and longevity programs. In particular, we wish to recognize Warren Taylor, whose enthusiasm, ceaseless hard work, and limitless patience has not only benefited the CR Society but also kept us going during an often trying writing process.

Iris Bass did an extraordinary job editing the manuscript, despite its arriving in disparate batches from all corners of the globe, and we thank our publisher, Matthew Lore of Da Capo/Perseus Books Group, for believing in this book through many reconceptions, revisions, and rewrites.

Michael Rae offered very useful scientific advice, and Al Pater helped us find obscure scientific literature.

Brian would like to thank Florence Banks for her patient support many, many years ago when he first took up writing. Lisa would like to thank Shree B. K. S. Iyengar for his brilliant contributions to yoga, which helped her maintain her health and equilibrium through her father's passing. For their efforts and contributions in the kitchen, Lisa thanks Peri Doslu, Jeff Pearlman, and Lynn Theard. And finally, for the brilliant blogging inspiration and the trials of being a CR goddess, Lisa thanks April Smith; Louise Gold for her stamina living on the roller coaster of being a woman on CR; and Peter Voss for his guidance in the formative stages of this book.

INDEX